WE LIVE IN
BUT KNOWLEDGE IS
DO YOU KNOW . . .

- How the clothes you send to the cleaners can expose you to high levels of carcinogens?

- Why housework can give you a headache?

- Why fast-food hamburgers can be deadly for a child?

- How cow's milk has been altered to pose a health risk to you?

- Why the new fat substitute is being called a "public health bomb"?

- How your skin may be telling you that your body is overloaded with toxins?

- How a special bath can stimulate feelings of sensuality and sexual responsiveness?

- How to create a wonderful wrinkle reducer from red wine?

- Which simple substance in apples can eliminate all toxins from your system?

FIND OUT IN . . .

TEN DAYS TO DETOX

TEN DAYS <u>TO</u> DETOX

How to Look and Feel a Decade Younger

Robin Westen

A DELL BOOK

Published by
Dell Publishing
a division of
Bantam Doubleday Dell Publishing Group, Inc.
1540 Broadway
New York, New York 10036

ISBN: 0-440-22513-2

Printed in the United States of America

Published simultaneously in Canada

March 1998

10   9   8   7   6   5   4   3   2   1
OPM

For Gabriel Sky,
who shows me the way

Special thanks to Howard Brofsky, Susan Lee Cohen, Terence and Anne Sellaro, Marilyn Buhlmann, Liza King, and all those who generously shared their stories.

Contents

Introduction

It's hard to ignore the signals when nature urges us to make a fresh start. We look in the mirror and suddenly see ourselves as though for the first time. Our complexion is lifeless, our eyes are without sparkle. We have little energy, and our creativity and drive seem always out of reach. At this crossroads we have a choice: to accept these conditions as our inevitable decline and continue existing without really experiencing the fullness of our lives or to stop the wheel, reverse the process, and thrill once more to life.

The choice may be obvious, but the solution is not simple. Unfortunately, there's no easy way to cleanse the body and spirit. One day of watching what you eat, or what you think, or randomly paying attention to potential toxins in your environment won't result in any permanent improvement. In order truly to change, you must not only become conscious of toxic conditions but maintain the will to seek out a purified state. *Ten Days to Detox* offers you a health-affirming program that is direct and powerful.

Mystics have always known the virtue of the number ten. In tarot cards ten is represented by the Wheel of Fortune. In the Kabbalah, the metaphysical system by which its students learn about God and the universe, ten is the number said to be boundless in origin and having no ending. According to the Kabbalah, this number also denotes a change in conditions and rules both the spiritual and scientific aspects of life. Astrologically viewed, ten rules the planet Uranus and, as in the Kabbalah, signifies change. Of course there are the Ten Commandments and, not to be "discounted," our ten fingers and ten toes. In numerology, the study of the occult significance of numbers, ten means "all." Similarly, the *Ten Days to Detox* program purifies *all* aspects of your being: the spiritual, physical, and emotional. The initial three days of the program are devoted to preparation, the following five to a cleansing "flush," and the final two days to balancing and reentry.

In the first section of the book you'll learn about the necessity of detoxing: how we are infused daily with harmful "antinutritional" contaminants like preservatives, sugar, caffeine, tobacco, processed yeast products, and artificial ingredients; how environmental toxins like free radicals, lead, pesticides, and carbon monoxide, as well as many ingredients in common household cleaners, rob us of our natural defenses against aging and illness. You'll read about the dangers that hide in many over-the-counter and commonly prescribed medications, along with those toxic ingredients that contaminate shampoos and other popular beauty products. You'll see how emotional toxins like stress, abusive relationships, and day-to-day contact with negative energy are stunningly detrimental. I cite numerous scientific studies from major medical journals, describing the relationship between toxins and such diseases as cancer, arthritis, diabetes, heart disease, and depression.

The book's next section offers a hands-on diagnostic questionnaire that will help you calculate the level of your toxicity and the main culprits. The questions are varied and touch all areas of your life. For example, how do the seasons affect your energy? Do certain people make you feel angry or sad when you are around them? How do specific flavors (spicy, sour, sweet) affect your appetite? Do you have a hard time sleeping? Do you frequently suffer with colds, stomachaches, insomnia, and/or headaches? The first step in eliminating toxins is to identify them, to become an observer, and to be open to the clues your body gives to its conditions and its needs. Did you know that dry skin, brittle nails and hair, weak muscle tone, even cellulite are signals of specific toxic conditions?

I'm confident that you'll find the questionnaire enlightening and accessible, but be prepared to allow time to consider each question and to calculate the results. The questionnaire covers diet, exercise, sleep, emotional imbalances, stress levels, family life, and childhood experiences, as well as a comprehensive look at your medical history. To establish an effective baseline, the diagnostic questionnaire is extensive, but the revelations make the investment in your time and concentration worth it. Once you have established your baseline, you'll be able to calculate the level of toxicity in your life, focus on its origin, and consider the remedies specifically suited for each one.

Next, *Ten Days to Detox* offers a realistic fasting schedule that enables you to cleanse your body by altering your diet and lifestyle. Throughout, there are references to studies that prove that detoxing methods like cleansing diets, lymphatic drainage massage, exercise, meditation, and saunas are powerful combatants against illness and premature aging. For example, you'll learn how diet may help prevent or cure various forms of cancer;

how exercise elevates moods, prevents disease, and cleanses the cells; how meditation, deep breathing, even keeping a bowl of salt water near an unpleasant companion can reduce the effects of emotionally draining and disease-causing vibrations.

You'll discover that what makes us toxic is not what happens to us in our lives but our mental and physical reactions to what comes into our lives. When you are unaware of your intrinsic wholeness, you can unwittingly invite disease by treating the body carelessly and by burdening your mind and nervous system with toxic thoughts and emotions. You can also abuse your system by repeatedly exposing it to environmental toxins, getting too little rest and exercise, pursuing too many damaging, unhappy relationships, and maintaining a toxic diet.

Since the food we eat today becomes the cells of our bodies tomorrow, *Ten Days to Detox* includes an extensive healing foods and vitamin, mineral, and herb guide. Foods and supplements that can cleanse particular organs and are especially helpful in dealing with specific diseases and emotional imbalances are described. For example, you'll learn that asparagus is valued for its diuretic qualities (cleanses kidneys and bladder) and possesses a high mineral content; that yarrow tea purifies the liver; and that rhubarb is remarkably rich in vitamins A and C as well as minerals, revitalizes the blood, regulates digestion, and sparks lackluster appetites. You'll discover that cucumbers have long been noted for improving the complexion, cleansing the liver, aiding in digestion, diabetes, and headaches as well as helping keep you "cool as a cucumber" in summer months.

But the detox program won't work without a firm commitment from you. Attitude is everything. You can feast on the facts, but first you need to bring your own silver tray, embracing the program not only in your mind but also in your heart.

During the ten-day period you will become aware of your perfect nature and begin to participate consciously in the healing process. You will discover the fundamental cause of your discomfort and unease and through a detoxification process reestablish an inner physical and emotional harmony. When you complete the program, you will have taken the final step in detoxing and healing: the acceptance of health.

You will also possess the unshakable conviction that nature's tendency is to heal, to regain and maintain the natural balance. This means you will stop anticipating illness, expecting sickness to overtake you tomorrow, next winter, in old age, or whenever. Anxiety itself creates the number one toxic trigger for disease. It sets in motion a circle in which inner negative expectations affect the outer circumstances, which in turn set off toxic responses in our physical and mental systems. By the conclusion of the detox program, you will have mastered the ability to recognize the interaction between your mind, emotions, and physical body.

Purified through detoxing, you can finally experience your true essence. You'll realize that you are not your sickness or imbalance. Your original nature is wholeness, health.

You are perfect, infinite, and glowing energy.

1

The Toxic Connection

*Past civilizations have been destroyed
by barbarians from outside, but we
are doing this job ourselves.*
—Malcolm Muggeridge

At twenty-nine Carla Evans could hardly walk a block without becoming winded, could not eat a meal before nausea, dizziness, and stomach cramps set in, or could barely get through the day without muscle tremors and a crippling fatigue. She told me that it felt as if she had the flu nearly every day of her life. Doctors told her otherwise. One after another they diagnosed their patient with "somatoform disorder," a polite way of saying it was "all in her head."

Finally a test specifically designed to break down blood chemistry, one rarely offered by orthodox physicians, revealed a different story.

Contaminating Carla's bloodstream were high levels of the chemicals DDT, trichloroethylene, and DDE. In other words, her body was something like a toxic swamp. Especially sensitive, and allergic to many common chemicals, Carla was suffering from environmental illness: Formaldehyde in shopping malls gave her headaches, car exhausts made her faint, and certain cleaning solvents sent her into near-suicidal depression.

The prescription for healing was strenuous. Besides a host of such treatments as acupuncture, deep tissue massage, weekly saunas, and a controlled diet, Carla removed all chemical cleaners, cosmetics, plastics, and irritating fabrics like thick synthetic rugs from her home. She also had six large dental cavities that had been filled over the years with mercury amalgam replaced with composite resin, a less toxic substance. With constant vigilance, Carla is finally on the way to recovery. Still, she must spend the rest of her life painstakingly avoiding toxic chemicals.

Although most of us are not as environmentally sensitive as Carla, no one is completely immune. When the total load of toxins exceeds the body's ability to deal with them, signs and symptoms of toxicity are evident in everyone's immune, endocrine, and gastrointestinal systems. Chemical toxins and other environmental stresses inevitably wear down the immune system until it can no longer protect itself completely from everyday irritants; airborne toxic substances travel through pathways in the nose and lead directly to the brain.

In recent history we've managed to change drastically the chemistry of our environment. In just one year 5,705,670,380 pounds of chemical pollutants are released into the environment we eat, breathe, and live in. The fact that we are seeing more and more people becoming sensitive to a dysfunctional degree may be because they have been steeped in this chemical environment since childhood.

On the following pages I'll describe the common toxins to which we are most frequently exposed during our daily lives. Although this material may seem hopelessly negative, perhaps overwhelming, take heart. The amount of time toxins stay in our bodies is directly related to the balance between the amount of exposure and the amount of detoxification and excretion. In other words, there's a way out.

Once you begin your journey of detoxification, the reversal process will be set in motion. You will no longer be a victim. One day you will be master of your body, master of your mind, and master of your self.

ENVIRONMENTAL ENEMIES

Dry Cleaning

We pay a price for looking neat and pressed—far beyond the cost of our dry cleaning bills. Dry cleaning involves soaking garments in harsh chemical solvents, including perchloroethylene, a highly toxic carcinogen that has been proved to cause harm to the central nervous system as well as most major organs. The National Institute for Occupational Safety and Health found that dry cleaning workers had significantly higher than average rates of cancers of the intestines, esophagus, and pancreas. Another study found that driving around for fifteen minutes with only three wool suits hanging in a car exceeds the maximum level of safe exposure to perchloroethylene by over 300 percent.

Formaldehyde

This chemical is found in a number of such household products as plywood, particleboard, furniture, carpets, some types of foam installation, no-iron bed linens, permanent press clothing, and polyester-cotton fabric. It can also be a by-product of combustion and may occur from using unvented appliances that burn fuel. At the very least, formaldehyde, a strong-smelling color-less gas, irritates eyes and causes sneezing, cough-ing, and skin irritation. Intense exposure can adversely affect our organs and has been shown to cause cancer in humans.

Radon Gas

Radon is a naturally occurring radioactive gas that may be emitted continually in some homes. Indoor radon levels vary with the amount of ra-dium in the surrounding soil and the house de-sign. Houses with poor ventilation or designs that encourage air and water to leak through the foun-dations are more susceptible to trapping radon. It has been proved that prolonged exposure to high levels of radon increases the risk of lung cancer.

Carbon Monoxide

Carbon monoxide in high concentration can cause dizziness, weakness, nausea, and disorienta-tion. These symptoms are often confused with the flu or food poisoning. But this type of indoor pol-lution is emitted by an improperly maintained heating system or any other unvented appliance that burns gas, oil, kerosene, or wood. Using these types of appliances frequently can increase exposure to this toxin. Very high levels of carbon monoxide can cause unconsciousness and lead to death.

Bacteria and Fungi

Bacteria and fungi affect the quality of indoor air and can be found in such sources as humidifiers, air conditioners, humans, and pets. In fact, humans and pets are actually sources of many bacterial and viral elements. Bacteria, fungi, and viruses can cause both common illnesses, such as influenza, and less common illnesses, such as Legionnaires' disease and humidifier fever.

Other Chemicals

If housework gives you a headache, it's not surprising. Ammonia, phenol, and other chemicals contained in common cleaning products, especially those with aerosol sprays, may be the culprits. These chemicals are especially toxic and can irritate the skin, eyes, nose, and throat as well as cause irregularities in the nervous system.

You might also get a toxic reaction trying to keep your hair clean. Most commercial shampoos contain at least one synthetic cleanser, or surfactant, that manufacturers include so they can deliver the burst of suds that consumers expect. While surfactants are considered safe by the Food and Drug Administration (FDA), these synthetics can carry the risk of serious chemical contamination. Many experts also advise avoiding laureth compounds (sodium laureth sulfate) or any other ingredients that include the syllable *eth*. These compounds are derivatives of natural coconut oil, but because of the way they're processed, they can be contaminated with a carcinogen called 1,4-dioxane that has been linked to cancer.

FOUL FOOD

Most of us choose to eat what tastes good to our personal palates, but too often our choices promote neither health nor well-being. In 1995, when the National Consumers League asked its members if they had once been a victim of food poisoning, 44 percent responded yes. Skin irritation, sluggishness, chronic constipation, impatience, and depression all are symptoms of food poisoning. Even foods that aren't tainted cause ill effects. Think about how you felt the last time you succumbed to a fast-food fix or finished off a bag of chips. Were you edgy? Depressed? Angry? Craving *more*? Sick to your stomach? Or . . . worse.

A few hours after Susan Kamp treated her daughter, Charlotte, to a burger in a fast-food restaurant in West Palm Beach, Florida, the five-year-old developed diarrhea. The next morning she was in pain, and by the end of the day Susan noticed a horrifying pool of blood beneath the child. She scooped her daughter into her arms and, with a pounding heart, drove to the hospital.

Charlotte's symptoms ranged from kidney failure to severe disorientation. The doctors suspected *E. coli* poisoning and began a treatment of detoxification with blood transfusions. After constant vigilance and prayers, by the tenth day of her hospitalization, Charlotte's condition finally improved. But doctors say because of the damage the bacteria caused to her kidneys, she will be at increased risk of kidney problems later in life, perhaps even in need of a transplant.

Charlotte's mother explained her horror to a reporter: "I can't tell you what it's like to sit at your child's bedside and have doctors not be able to look you in the eye and tell you whether your daughter will live or die . . . just because you fed her a hamburger."

E. Coli

Illness-producing bacteria have become the leading cause of acute kidney failure among children in the United States, causing some 40,000 illnesses and 250 to 500 deaths each year. According to a team of researchers at Tufts University in Boston, as much as 25 percent of the ground meat sold in our supermarkets may contain bacteria that are capable of causing kidney failure and related complications. Unrinsed fruits and vegetables can also be breeding grounds for bacteria. Some outbreaks of illness caused by *E. coli* have been linked beyond burgers to lettuce and other produce exposed to fecal matter during growing or transport to the supermarket.

Seafood

To avoid the devastating damage of *E. coli* as well as of high levels of cholesterol, many of us choose fish instead of red meat. But contaminated seafood causes at least fifty thousand and possibly one hundred thousand people to become ill each year, mostly from bacteria and naturally occurring toxins, according to the Center for Disease Control (CDC). Tropical or island water fish such as snapper and grouper, as well as bluefish, mahimahi, and fresh tuna, are highest in natural toxins.

Additionally, according to the Center for Science in the Public Interest, many fish exposed to chemical toxins from industrial waste have made it into our food chain, despite stringent laws to protect the consumer.

Pesticides

Unfortunately, we're not guaranteed a healthy diet even when we eat so-called nutritious foods like fruits, nuts, and vegetables. A major study conducted by the National Academy of Sciences notes that these foods are among those most likely to contain residues of pesticides. Another study conducted by the Environmental Working Group, an advocacy organization in Washington, D.C., found that more than 80 percent of peach, apple, and celery samples contained residues of one or more pesticides. The group listed twenty-one different chemicals that are used on apples alone.

Although it often takes time for the harmful effects of these toxins to take their toll, some experts warn that subtle damage from toxins early in life can lead to problems such as cancer, reproductive abnormalities, and hormonal irregularities later on.

Genetically Engineered Hormones

Despite those white mustaches seen on smiling celebrity faces in milk advertisements, the controversy over hormonally treated cows continues. According to the FDA and other major scientific organizations, the genetically engineered hormone (RbST), used to treat cows so they will increase their milk production, is one of the most stringently researched animal drugs the agency has ever reviewed. Still, the Consumers Union and other groups say that there are serious problems. Some studies, for example, have found that treated cows have a higher rate of mastitis, which is routinely treated with antibiotics that could, at the least, get into a milk drinker's body and boost resistance to bacteria-fighting drugs.

Bacillus Cereus

The bacterial strain *Bacillus cereus* is present in a wide variety of foods, including meat, poultry, and starchy foods like noodles. Fried rice stands out as a leading cause in the United States of vomiting-accompanied foodborne illness from *Bacillus cereus*; scientists suspect it's because this food is often left out and then reheated before eating. All cooked leftovers should be refrigerated within two hours of serving. Even seemingly innocuous items like pasta or vegetables that have been left out for hours after cooking and then reheated down the line can bring on the debilitating symptoms of foodborne illness.

Food Additives and Preservatives

Sometime in the mid-sixties breweries in Quebec began putting increased amounts of a chemical called cobalt sulfate into beer. The additive had been used for several years to make the foam last longer. But over the next six months forty-eight beer drinkers became ill—and twenty died. Could such a tragedy happen again? Probably.

Although ingredient lists are right there on packages, many of the words are difficult or impossible to decipher. They include sodium stearoyl lactylate, an additive that keeps oil and water from separating in bread, and calcium propionate, an ingredient that prevents the growth of molds, bacteria, and other microorganisms and helps foods have a longer shelf life. Although most food additives do not cause toxic reactions, several do.

Joseph Maga, a professor of food science and human nutrition and the head of the Food Research and Development Center at Colorado State University, cites sulfites (found in dry fruits and wine) as a serious danger for an estimated 2 to 5 percent of the population. Many consumers have reported problems like severe headaches, nausea, and disorientation.

Since 1958 the FDA has been monitoring food additives, but many additives are still in our foods even though research trials have shown they cause cancer in rats. In fact, the Center for Science in the Public Interest suggests that certain additives should be avoided because they have been linked to birth defects, cancer, or other adverse reactions. CSPI's list includes:

Numerous food dyes
Brominated vegetable oil (BVO)
Butylated hydroxanisole (BHA)
Saccharin
Sodium nitrite/nitrate
Sulfur dioxide
Sodium bisulfite

Not only are these several of the most questionable additives, but many are used primarily in foods of low nutritional value.

Deserving special attention is monosodium glutamate (MSG), a powerful flavor enhancer capable of transforming the blandest food into a taste sensation. Adding MSG to processed food reduces the need for fresh, more flavorful ingredients. It has been used in Chinese restaurants for decades. But scientific findings show that a percentage of the population suffers from MSG symptom complex. The symptoms include headache; a burning sensation in the back of the neck, forearms, and chest; numbness in the back of the neck that radiates to the arms and back; tingling, warmth, and weakness in the face, temples, upper back, neck, and arms; facial pressure or tightness; chest pain; nausea; rapid heartbeat; drowsiness; and weakness.

Olestra

After twenty-five years and more than two hundred million dollars' worth of study and research, the Food and Drug Administration has recently approved the use of olestra, a so-called fat-free fat. Procter & Gamble, the company introducing the synthetic fat in its snack foods, says the safety of its product is backed up by 150,000 pages of data that include 150 studies and 45 clinical trials. P & G insists olestra is safe for consumers. But the reason olestra isn't fattening is that it cannot be digested; it passes straight through the body and out. The potentially fatal catch-22 is that a portion of the fat-soluble nutrients consumed at the same meal will attach themselves to olestra and exit the body along with it.

Drs. Walter Willett and Meir Stamfer of the Harvard School of Public Health, in a letter signed by twenty-five other health professionals, argue: "There is strong reason to suspect that the effects on the body from olestra will include increases in cancer, heart disease, stroke and blindness." Michael Jacobson of the Center for Science in the Public Interest calls olestra a "public health bomb."

High-Fat Diets

In an article published in *Science News* (June 1996), Janet Raloff writes that just the *taste* of fat has been shown to elevate blood levels of triglycerides in our bodies. This is surprising information, although the devastating effects of fatty diets on our cardiovascular systems is by now common knowledge. A high-fat diet is a one-way ticket to clogged arteries, heart disease, anticholesterol medications, angioplasty, or bypass surgery.

Less known, however, is the destructive effect high-fat diets may have on our eyesight. Researchers who conducted a survey of more than two thousand people (between the ages of forty-five and eighty-five) found that those who reported eating the most saturated fat had an 80 percent greater chance of developing early degeneration of the retina (called age-related macular degeneration) than those who said they ate the least. Although there's no definitive answer for why fats are associated with the disease, scientists suggest that just as too much fat can clog the arteries to the heart, it may also clog the vessels

15

leading to the eyes, thereby reducing the flow of nutrient-rich blood.

The link between high cholesterol levels and ovarian cancer has also been studied. Researchers found that women with the highest cholesterol levels were more than three times as likely to get ovarian cancer as were women with the lowest cholesterol levels.

PHARMACEUTICALS

Illness and deaths directly related to the use of conventional prescription drugs should be considered one of the leading diseases in the United States, scientists wrote in *Archives of Internal Medicine*. Annually these drugs cost the economy more than $75 billion (an amount that could feed twenty million Americans for a year) and up to $136 billion when loss of productivity is included. More than 28 percent of all hospital admissions are from drug-related illness, resulting in nine million hospitalizations a year.

"Most conventional drugs are intended to relieve pain and discomforts as quickly as possible. And they often do this," says Dr. Joseph E. Pizzorno, the president of Bastyr University in Seattle and the author of *An Encyclopedia of Natural Medicine*. "However, the problem with this approach is that these medications do not promote health. And worse, they allow the underlying cause to remain and the illness to progress."

Antacids

Millions of us who suffer "heartburn" or acid indigestion take acid-neutralizing pills bought over the counter. Until recently antacids were the most common drug for this ailment. Now drugs like Tagamet (or h2 blockers), which were once only prescription items, are being sold over the counter. Some believe that drugs like Tagamet pose potential health risks because they interfere with the stomach's normal production of acid.

Cold Medications

Although many Americans reach for relief from their common cold by taking aspirin, acetaminophen, and decongestants, research shows they should think twice. For example, a high dose of acetaminophen can potentially cause dangerous liver-damaging effects. Some decongestants contain drugs that may cause hypertension, restlessness and agitation. Topical nasal decongestants, if used for more than three days in a row, may lead to what is termed "rebound congestion." This happens when, after an individual discontinues using the drug, the congestion actually becomes worse than it was originally. Finally, while some cold medications may relieve the symptoms of a cold, none will cure the cold.

Synthetic Estrogens for Menopause

The conventional way to treat menopause symptoms is with an animal-source estrogen or a synthetic estrogen, usually a drug called Premarin. But substantial research now documents the potential side effects—fluid retention, weight gain, irritability, postmenopausal bleeding, migraine headaches, hypertension—and the increased risk of breast and uterine cancers.

Weight-Loss Products

We spend about six billion dollars a year on weight-loss products and diet plans. Nonetheless, in the past decade the average American adult has gained ten pounds. Both nonprescription drugs (such as phenylpropanolamine and benzocaine) and prescription drugs (such as amphetamines) promote weight loss, but their results are generally only temporary. In fact, studies show that individuals who use these drugs rapidly regain their weight losses because the underlying cause of the weight gain is not addressed.

Cortisone Cream for Eczema

About 5 percent of the population suffers with eczema, a common skin irritation. Cortisone cream is frequently prescribed for eczema, taken either in a prescription form or in over-the-counter products. Although this treatment alleviates the severe itching (one of the symptoms of eczema), it does not treat the root of the disease. Inevitably, once the treatment stops, the condition returns. Moreover, long-term use of cortisone may cause several potential side effects, from local thinning of the skin and increased susceptibility to infection to suppression of the adrenal glands.

DENTAL CARE

Mercury

The most common dental material used in our teeth is known as amalgam, a soft composite used to fill cavities. It's an alloy of two or more metals, including a trace of zinc, copper (6 percent), tin (9 percent), silver (35 percent), and mercury (50 percent). More than one hundred years ago the American Society of Dental Surgeons required its members to sign "pledges" promising not to use it in dental fillings out of concern for mercury's danger.

Even back then, however, the safety of mercury was strongly debated. In fact, internal strife over the safety of mercury was one of the causes leading to the creation in 1859 of the American Dental Association (ADA) whose leaders did not oppose the use of mercury. Today it is estimated that more than a hundred million mercury fillings are placed in the mouths of dental patients each year.

Yet scientific evidence strongly suggests that mercury amalgams are a major source of toxic mercury exposure. As long as you have mercury fillings, you inhale mercury vapor twenty-four hours a day. Because mercury is a heavy metal, it acts as a free radical, which is a highly reactive, charged particle that can cause damage to body tissues if inhaled or absorbed. When present in excess, heavy metals can block enzymes necessary for the body's detoxification process.

Mercury toxicity has been shown to contribute to kidney malfunctions, cardiovascular diseases, neuropsychological problems, reproductive disorders, and birth defects. Symptoms of mercury toxicity include anorexia, depression, swollen glands, insomnia, moodiness, memory loss, nausea, diarrhea, gum decay, headaches, and fatigue.

Dental Sealants

A study at Spain's University of Granada determined that the plastic resins frequently used by dentists since 1965 to seal out bacteria and repair teeth may be leaching into saliva and body tissues at a dangerous rate. When the scientists applied a conventional amount of dental sealant to the molars of eighteen volunteers, they found that between 90 to 931 micrograms of bisphenol-A (the sealant's main ingredient) leached into the patient's saliva within one hour after treatment. Once it enters the body, bisphenol-A can imitate the natural hormone estrogen, producing seriously harmful effects, such as contributing to breast cancer and affecting the reproductive system of fetuses. Evidence also suggests that bisphenol-A may leach into saliva for up to two years following its placement.

TOXIC EMOTIONAL REACTIONS

It is not the actual events in our lives but our *reaction* to the events that create stress, anger, guilt, envy, and other emotional pain. If we can somehow just see that everything is in flux, that we are truly not what is happening to us, and that life is a journey with lessons that are benevolent, we would be able to sail above adversity, stay healthy, clear, and joy-filled.

A tough challenge. Still, most of us in our quiet moments can understand this message and reflect upon its deep and universal truth. If we can stay involved in life yet allow our negative emotions to remain detached, we have the potential to be happy with bodies that reflect our state of contentment.

Stress

The mind-body connection has been recognized since ancient times. Now researchers at the American Institute of Stress, a New York–based not-for-profit organization, maintain that 75 to 90 percent of patients' visits to physicians are for ailments that have some kind of link with stress.

Stress begins in the brain with perceptions of and emotions about a particular external event and ends up in the body as aches and pains, fatigue, headaches, heart palpitations, high blood pressure, stomach ailments, uneven breathing, hives, psoriasis, weight gain (or loss), or a host of other less common but more serious illnesses.

As Dr. Redford Williams says in his book *Anger Kills,* the brain under stress signals the adrenal glands to produce cortisol and adrenaline, which are responsible for most of the physical symptoms of stress. The part of your body that experiences the stress is usually the weakest link in your system. You probably know what it is; it always acts up when you're under stress. But no part of the body escapes these stress chemicals; in excess they destroy the inner linings of arteries, increase water and salt retention, stimulate blood clotting, reduce infection-fighting T cells, and affect blood circulation and muscle reactivity. These changes in turn may affect hair and nail growth, gum health, respiration, and digestion. They also affect menstruation and fertility; several studies have shown that the stress of infertility interferes with the release of hormones that can regulate ovulation. In one study 3 percent of women with fertility problems became pregnant within six months after they had learned to reduce their stress levels.

Physical stress occurs when an external or natural change or force acts upon the body. Extreme heat or cold, overwork, injuries, malnutrition, and exposure to drugs and poisons are examples of physical stress. Physical and emotional stress can overlap, as in special body conditions, such as pregnancy, menopause, adolescence, and aging. During these times body metabolism is increased or lowered, changing the body's physical functions, which in turn affect one's mental and emotional outlook on life. A certain amount of stress is useful as a motivating factor, but when it occurs in excess or is of the wrong kind, the effect is detrimental.

If there is no outlet for stress, then the body must react to it by channeling physical reactions inward to one of the organ systems, such as the digestive, circulatory, or nervous system. The system reacts adversely, and ulcers, hypertension, backache, atherosclerosis, allergic reactions, asthma, fatigue, or insomnia can develop.

Anxiety, a fearful or distressful feeling, is responsible for the stress many of us experience. Anything that threatens a person's body, job, loved ones, or values may cause anxiety. If you cannot cope with a situation, stress on the body is increased, resulting in many of the disorders associated with stress. The increase in the production of adrenal hormones that occurs with stress raises the metabolism of protein, fats, and carbohydrates producing instant energy for the body to use. As a result of this increased metabolism, there is an increased excretion of protein, potassium, and phosphorus and a decreased storage of calcium. Many stress-related disorders are not the direct result of the stress itself but the result of nutrient deficiencies caused by increased metabolic rate during periods of stress. For example, vitamin C is utilized by the adrenal gland during stressful conditions, and sufficiently severe or prolonged stress will cause a depletion of vitamin C in the tissues.

Anger

According to Redford, here's what happens to your body when you're angry: Aggressive thoughts percolate in your cerebral cortex, sending out a wake-up call to a group of hypothalamic nerve cells deeper within the brain. These cells in turn send messages even farther down in the base of your brain, where they cause outgoing nerves to signal the adrenal glands sitting on top of the kidneys to pump large doses of both adrenaline and cortisol into your bloodstream. As the adrenaline reaches your heart, it begins to pound faster and faster and your blood pressure rises. At the same time, the activated hypothalamic emergency center stimulates sympathetic nerves to constrict the arteries carrying blood to your skin, kidney, and intestines. Eventually the adrenaline causes your arteries to open wide.

The result? You feel a pounding heart, sweaty palms, and deep, rapid breathing. What you don't feel is that the adrenaline is silently stimulating your fat cells to empty their contents into your bloodstream and that your liver is converting the fat into cholesterol. The excess cholesterol is absorbed into the artery.

Five years down the road, if you're still experiencing frequent bouts of anger, a clot may form and life-sustaining blood will no longer be able to pass through your arteries to nourish your heart muscle. A portion of the blood-starved heart muscles will die. If this happens, you will become one of the five hundred thousand–plus Americans who has a heart attack that year.

On the emotional level, countless studies show that uncontrolled anger impairs relationships, and a considerable body of research acknowledges the negative impact of poor social interaction. For several years, for example, Dr. George Kaplan and his colleagues followed thousands of healthy residents of Alameda County, California. Those residents who had the fewest social ties had higher death rates than those people who maintained close, satisfying relationships. Further, married men live longer than bachelors, and additional research shows married cancer patients tend to live longer than unmarried cancer patients.

Because hostile people are likely to be more socially isolated than their less angry counterparts, a lack of social support is one pathway to disease for hostile people, but it remains to be shown how social isolation harms health. One possibility is that people lacking social ties are less apt to have good health habits and may not seek medical attention in a timely way or remember to take prescription drugs, eat healthy diets, or take vitamin supplements. There's also no one around to encourage a smoker to quit.

Social isolation caused by anger may also impose increased stress that may have harmful biological consequences. Andrew Baum, a psychologist, found that among people living near the Three Mile Island nuclear facility in Pennsylvania after the 1979 accident, those reporting lower levels of social support excreted higher levels of stress hormones in their urine. Conversely, having a confidant with whom to share concerns could reduce the biological impact of disease.

Insecurity, Envy, and Jealousy

If we are insecure even when we have abundance, we are in effect investing our energy in the fear of future want. Our habit of comparing what we have now with what others possess produces this sense of insecurity, which denies us the capacity to enjoy what we have already. It is a kind of addiction that brings anxiety and drives us to amass more than we need. With this mental addiction of achieving a sense of security through possession of more and more things, we no longer remember what we originally meant by "more."

The word "more" is all right, but how much more? "Security" is always a relative term, and it seems just always out of reach.

It's true that we all differ on how much we are in control of our emotions and how much of our emotions are in control of us. The balance is partly determined by factors of temperament (often inherited), partly by a phenomenon that psychologists call level of arousal, partly by training, and partly by experience. In order to reach an emotional equilibrium, you have to recognize the strength of your emotions and exert a reasonable degree of awareness over them, making sure your emotional responses are relevant to the situation and not being driven by jealousy, envy, or insecurity. When jealousy, envy, and insecurity pervade our thoughts, every aspect of our physical and emotional well-being is adversely affected in the same way stress and anger damage our health.

Depression

Chronic states of sadness, including bleak expectations for the future, may make the organs in your body susceptible to a host of serious illnesses. Researchers at Duke University tracked heart disease and mood symptoms in 730 men and women over age twenty-seven and found that people with symptoms of depression, such as hopelessness and low self-esteem, were 70 percent more likely to have heart attacks than those whose outlooks were cheerier. Researchers suspect that depression may disrupt nerves that relax the blood vessels. It is also possible that depressed people have stickier platelets, the blood cells involved in clotting. This might mean that depressed people have blood that clots more easily, a condition that can lead to heart attacks because clots can block blood vessels leading to the heart.

Another study that traced people thirteen years after they had been screened for depression found that those who were depressed were four times as likely to have a heart attack as those with more upbeat attitudes. The study, conducted by Dr. William W. Eaton of the Johns Hopkins School of Hygiene and Public Health, included 1,551 persons living in the Baltimore area who had taken part in a survey in the early 1980s documenting depression in the general population. Those who had been depressed or suffered symptoms of manic depression thirteen years earlier were almost twice as likely to suffer heart attacks. In contrast, just 37 of the 1,107 subjects who had not suffered depression when the study began had heart attacks in the intervening years.

Depression in fact harms more women than does AIDS or cancer. In 1990 suicide was the number one cause of death and disability for women ages fifteen to forty-four worldwide. By the year 2020 it will rank second only to heart disease, the world's leading cause of death and disability for men and women of all ages, according to the prediction of a five-year study by the World Health Organization, the World Bank, and the Harvard School of Public Health.

Hopelessness also exhibits a strong statistical link with the emergence of new cases of cancer. Moreover, the link holds up regardless of the presence of other major risk factors for disease and death, including cigarette smoking, high blood pressure, alcohol use, and lack of social support. Scientists surmise that hopeless people may experience surges of stress hormones, which can undermine the heart and other internal organs, or they may undergo immune changes leading to cancer. Not surprisingly, other research indicates that optimism in the face of losses and failures promotes mental and physical health.

Many people accept depression as a natural condition of life, but it is not. Look over the questions below.* If you answer yes to many of these questions, there's a good chance that you are suffering at least some symptoms of depression. Feel

* Source: Dr. William Eaton/Johns Hopkins University.

confident that the detox program can help you see the flickering light at the end of the tunnel.

- In your lifetime, have you ever had two weeks or more when nearly every day you felt sad, blue, or depressed?
- Has there ever been a period of two weeks or longer when you lost your appetite?
- Have you ever lost weight without trying to— as much as two pounds a week for several weeks or as much as ten pounds altogether?
- Have there ever been at least two weeks when you had an increase in appetite? Did your eating increase so much that you gained as much as two pounds a week for several weeks or ten pounds altogether?
- Have you ever had two weeks or more when nearly every night you had trouble falling asleep, staying asleep, or waking too early?
- Have you ever had two weeks or more when nearly every morning you would wake up at least two hours before you wanted to?
- Have you ever had two weeks or longer when nearly every day you were sleeping too much?

BEFORE MOVING ON

Check your mental state. After you have read how we are not only bombarded by environmental pollutants created by technology but affected by negative thoughts we create in our own minds, it's natural to feel a sense of hopelessness. *Let go of those feelings.* Trust that you will be given everything needed to change your life and begin anew. Have faith in yourself and in your desire to change.

> *Create a castle of positivity around you; it will offer protection from those arrows of negativity.*

2

Come Clean, Change Your Life

A monk came to Joshu and asked,
"What is the meaning of Zen?"
The Master replied, "Have you eaten your breakfast?"
"Yes," said the monk, "I have eaten."
"Then wash your bowl," said Joshu.
At that instant the monk was enlightened.
—from The Little Book of Zen Wisdom

The first time I tried to detox, more than a decade ago, I was certain that I could never get through it. In fact, I didn't. Three hours into the regimen I was sneaking handfuls of chips and later in the day stopping by the corner store for a bar of chocolate. Instead of feeling better, I felt awful. Not only had I blown the diet, but I felt weak, a victim to my cravings. In those days I had a terrible attitude. I wanted to achieve results without any effort. I wanted a miracle.

Several months later I tried another purification program. This time I knew that it would take some strong inner work. When that little voice said, "Oh, go ahead and have a handful of chips. How much difference will it make?" I knew what to tell myself: "Plenty!" Instead of strolling around my kitchen, I walked in the woods. I meditated on change rather than the sweetness of melting chocolate. I kept quiet, turned inward, and steadfastly continued on my path.

Two days into my fast I began to feel more alive, and by the third day I was in a state of utter exhilaration. When the detox concluded, my life had changed. Stress, random thoughts, impatience, unhappiness, body fatigue, and stiffness drained away. For the first time in my adult life I was truly at peace with a clear, uncritical mind and an open, loving heart. I learned that miracles *do* happen, but I had to be prepared, ready to receive.

CURING DISEASE

Joel Fuhrman, a New Jersey physician and the author of *Fasting and Eating for Health,* says he's seen the miracle of fasting through his own experience with patients. According to Fuhrman, supervised detox fasting has helped cure his patients of numerous diseases, including digestive problems, lupus, migraine headaches, hypertension, diabetes, asthma, heart disease, and arthritis. "Detoxing should be seen as a legitimate alternative to undergoing medical procedures," says Fuhrman. "Any person with high blood pressure or coronary artery disease could choose to take medication for the rest of their life, or go into a fasting program and quickly obliterate the need."

Many of Fuhrman's patients, like Richard Descond, have turned to curative detoxing as a last resort. When Descond was forty-six, his lifestyle was taking a serious toll. Not only was he severely overweight thanks to a diet of fast food, but he was also experiencing excruciating headaches, achy bones, and stomach problems. When he could no longer ignore his symptoms, he made an appointment with his physician. After a thorough battery of tests Descond was diagnosed with bone cancer and told he had fewer than five years to live. Pushed to take action, he finally accepted responsibility for his health. He went on a strict, supervised forty-day fast. Today he is free of bone cancer. His immune system is strong; he is healthier than he has been in more than two decades.

Dr. Elson Haas, a general practitioner, the director of the Preventative Medical Center of Marin in San Rafael, California, and the author of *A Diet for All Seasons,* also reports on the healing effects of a detox fast. "During a fast, the immune system is spared the extra work of dealing with common allergens like wheat, milk, eggs, coffee, yeast and corn. Instead, the immune system is free to produce new disease-fighting cells and antibodies. Many of my patients have beaten serious illnesses including viral infections."

Even for those fortunate enough to be in optimal health, detox fasting is beneficial; it gives your body a much-deserved break. During a fast you reduce the amount of energy and attention the body needs to spend on digestion. Instead your body's energy can focus on eliminating built-up wastes and toxins. As a result of this expulsion, the mind is elevated to a higher level. You're given the ability to perceive subtler aspects of your being.

In an article for *Fitness* magazine, journalist Ben Napp describes his mental state after the third day of a fasting regimen: "It was as if I were a windowpane that had just been wiped so clean the sun could shine in with full force and brilliance. All food then seemed like specks of dust that would block the full effects of its energizing rays."

LOOKING YOUNGER

Besides helping the mind and body return to a more balanced and functional state, detoxing will restore radiant youthfulness. Most people perceive skin flaws as mere cosmetic problems, but blemishes are the skin's way of working overtime to eliminate toxins. As wastes accumulate, eliminative organs work harder to keep pace. The liver, kidneys, and colon are the ordinary channels of elimination. If they become overloaded, the body resorts to other means of elimination—lungs, reproductive tract, skin, eyes, nose, and other mucous membranes—in an attempt to clean itself.

Skin disorders, poor coloring, or uneven tone and texture may be the body's way of saying it's overloaded with wastes. Puffy or swollen eyes, dark circles under the eyes, crusty or mucus formations in the eyes, bad breath or morning breath, water retention in the skin, and such skin disorders as psoriasis, eczema, dermatitis, and seborrhea all indicate that a person's skin and body want a well-deserved rest.

Even if you have no obvious skin problems, your skin can profit from a detoxing fast. The natural glow returns to the face as capillary circulation and lymphatic drainage improve; blemishes, blotches, and spots diminish or disappear; in the eyes redness lessens, whites become whiter, and dark circles disappear; skin texture appears smoother and softer; and sometimes fine lines fade. Accelerating the exfoliation of skin cells—the concept behind expensive skin treatments such as Retin-A and alpha hydroxy acids—occurs naturally during a fast. The body also generates new skin cells more rapidly. Exfoliation and cell renewal form the foundation for a fresh, youthful appearance.

Another key component of healthy skin is hydration, which means maintaining adequate moisture levels within the body. Drinking water is not enough to assure hydration. When you're dehydrated, your cells lack water while the areas between the cells retain too much water. Outwardly this shows up as puffiness, fluid retention, bloating, and poorly defined facial features. A detoxing fast eliminates the water trapped between the cells and allows freshwater to go into the cells, leaving your face and body with a more sculpted, youthful appearance.

MAKING A COMMITMENT

> *Life begets life.*
> *Energy creates energy.*
> *It is by spending oneself*
> *that one becomes rich.*
> —*Sarah Bernhardt*

You may be convinced that a detox program is exactly what you need to improve your life, but choosing this path isn't without its obstacles. The first two days of a detoxing program are the most difficult. During this time the body and mind crave old habits. Therefore, it's important to make a deep-rooted commitment *before* you begin your detox program; even with careful preparations and good intentions, hidden negative thoughts and blocks can prevent a detox program from being successful. We may think we want to change the way we are, but unconsciously we're resisting the idea.

Deep down, many of us don't believe change is really possible. To implement change in ourselves, we first need to become conscious of and explore these hidden resistances. The best way to conquer blocks that limit our potential and fuel our will to fail is to find them, explore them, and then root them out.

The following techniques will help in the process.

Journal Writing

Starting a journal a few days prior to embarking on the program is a good method for reinforcing your commitment. Write down those aspects of your physical and emotional life that you think need improvement. Be honest in projecting how difficult you believe it will be for you to stick to the regimen. Also, let yourself envision how you will feel when you do successfully detox. What changes will you experience in the way you look? The way you feel? The way you conduct your life? The way others relate to you? Be truthful when you write down your reactions, fears, and desires.

Psychologist Melanie Greenberg asked one group of college students to write detailed essays about a personal trauma, ranging from abuse to rape, and another set to write fictional accounts. Greenberg found that the students who had composed accurate accounts of their personal tribulations made two-thirds fewer trips to the doctor than the group that wrote fictional or impersonal accounts. Writing openly, Greenberg suggests, may help us develop a sense of control over our emotions, and this in turn may contribute to good health.

Affirmations, biblical proverbs, poems, excerpts from stories, and song lyrics have special significance for me during times of change, and I include these in my journal. If you're a visually connected individual, you may decide to draw, or cut out images and paste them in your notebook; these will inspire you along your journey. In any case, make your journal a reflection of your personal desire to change, and use it as a safe place to go during quiet or difficult times. Know that it is your private possession. Do not suggest others read your journal. Even if it's a symbolic gesture, there is a reason why many diaries are designed with locks and keys.

Dream Analysis

Dreams may provide clues to emotional problems and health difficulties months before danger signs show up on medical tests. Some scientists now believe that health-related, or prodromic, dreams occur when the body's cells detect minor chemical abnormalities and send warning signals through the nerves to the brain. The subconscious mind, which is much more adept at picking up these signals than the conscious mind, then expresses them in the form of dreams.

Learn to read the signals. If you dream of being hit on the head, it may mean you've got a migraine coming on; if you dream about someone changing a flat tire or putting out a fire, your body may be fighting an infection; if you're allergic to cats and you suddenly begin dreaming that you're petting one, you may be developing an allergy to something else. Dreams of collapsing houses, intruders, or ambushes can also be signs of illness.

As for positive dreams, newness, flowers, and housecleaning often represent returning to health. As you fall asleep, hold one of these images in your mind. Programming yourself to dream about health will send healing messages to your body and mind and ultimately enrich the detoxing process.

When you wake up in the morning, record in your journal what you dreamed and the emotions you experienced. This will help you note a potential health problem, so you can take steps to cure it during the detoxing process.

In a book that I found very helpful, *The Sensual Body*, Lucy Lidell suggests the following exercises:

Mirror

Most of the time we stop to look at our reflections only to see if we appear presentable. If we do pause in front of the mirror, it is often to criticize ourselves for the way we look rather than merely to observe or admire what we see. In the mirror gazing exercise you simply look at yourself naked in a mirror for approximately fifteen minutes, in order to learn to accept yourself and develop the same loving relationship with your own body that you would wish to have with a lover. It is important that you regard yourself compassionately, without judgment, just as you would look at a small child or a close friend. You may find this hard to do initially or may get drawn into criticizing aspects of yourself you wish were different.

Gazing at your reflection may also awaken memories or feelings of sadness or loneliness. Simply register whatever thoughts or feelings arise. They all are part of the process of getting to know and love yourself a little better, and it is only by expressing and accepting your feelings that you can begin to make a change.

Stretching

Look at a cat when it wakes up from sleep. It will move part of its body, pause, then move another part, until the whole body appears to be moved from within. This spontaneous stretching is one of the most fundamental ways of being totally present and eliminating physical resistance in the body.

Vital Stretching

You can provide the stimulus for vital stretching by lying down with your back on the floor, then slightly shifting your position or by rubbing or stretching yourself. Simply allow the movements to happen without directing them, and notice the sequence of sensations in your whole being. The impulse to move may be very slight or may increase unexpectedly, and it will vary from day to day. Good times to explore this vital stretch are when you wake up or after you've been sitting for a long time in one position.

Spine Stretch

Another simple stretch to release obstacles in the spine (where energy flows) involves lying on your back for ten minutes without moving. Imagine your spine elongating; envision a space between each vertebra filled with a clear white light. Next, slowly pull your left knee to your chest, hold for five seconds, and lower. Repeat with your right knee. Now pull up both knees, and hold for eight seconds. Return both legs to the floor, and remain supine. This time envision the white light from your spine making a cloud around your whole body. Feel your weightlessness and freedom. When your body is relaxed, you may slowly roll over and gently stand up. Lift your arms to the heavens, and then exhale while you bring them down to your side.

Breathing

Few people are aware of the powerful connection between breath and their emotions. Whenever we experience fear or discomfort, joy or excitement, we hold our breath. In fact, our emotions are so closely linked with breath that we can actually change how we feel by changing how we breathe.

In the spiritual traditions of many Eastern cultures, breath is believed to carry the life force or vital energy, known as prana, chi, and ki. In yoga, pranayama or the regulation of prana through breathing exercises is one of the principal daily practices. Pranayama not only energizes the whole body but also creates emotional stability and great clarity of mind.

Letting Go

Sit on the floor or a chair with your palms on your stomach. Slowly breathe in from your diaphragm to a count of seven; now release your breath slowly while pressing your fingers gently into your stomach. Move your fingers clockwise to a nearby spot on your stomach, and press firmly while repeating the breathing exercise. Continue moving your fingers and repeating the exercise until you've made a circle with your fingers.

BREATHING IN/ BREATHING OUT

Sit on the floor with your arms at chest level, fingers interlocked and palms facing outward. Breathing from your diaphragm, inhale deeply for seven seconds, and bring the backs of your hands in to touch your chest. Holding the inhalation, slowly release breath from your diaphragm, stretching your palms straight out in front of you. Imagine you're squeezing out all the air from your body through your fingertips. Hold for as long as you possibly can. Repeat the breathing in and breathing out exercises alternately seven times.

ALTERNATE BREATHING

Sit comfortably cross-legged on the floor or in a straight-backed chair. Close the right nostril by pinching it, and breathe in slowly through the left. When you have taken a full breath, close both nostrils for as long as is comfortable; then, keeping the left nostril closed, exhale slowly through the right. Now inhale through the right nostril, hold, and exhale through the left. Do this up to ten times.

Studying Self

To reach a goal, whatever it may be, it is necessary to remain single-minded in our effort, although the mind will no doubt tempt us to go in a hundred different directions. To move toward growth requires the persistent study of one's self. How do you study the self? Simply by asking, "What is a person? Who am I?" Stop identifying with those things that society has given you, like your name and title, or with such concepts as success or failure, beauty or ugliness. These are after all only relative values.

Concepts are not absolutes; they are all your own projections. They keep you revolving around the periphery of life and prevent you from coming in touch with the core of your being. Go beyond them and ask, "Who am I really? Who is moving? Who is eating? Who is meeting? Who is doing all these things?" The fundamental question is this: Who am I?

When we seriously ask this question, we become aware of the conflict between what we have been taught to think we ought to be and what we really are. It begins to dawn on us that we have not been living correctly. That is when we turn inward to discover the exact nature of our bodies, our minds, and, finally, the inside dwellers that are our true selves.

Positive Thinking

According to Brahma Kumaris, "What we say, what we do, what we feel—all have their origin in the mind. The energy of the human mind is thought. It is possibly one of the greatest but least understood resources of the universe." As more Western scientists look to the East for answers, they are agreeing that our states of mind do indeed affect our health, physically and emotionally, and that our expectations, attitudes, and emotions can make us sick or help us recover from illness and addictions.

Today psychoneuroimmunology—the study of the interactions of the brain's system of neurochemicals with the endocrine system of hormones and the immune system's defenses against infections—is a growing field. Sheldon Cohen, a psychologist at Carnegie-Mellon University, collected data from a five-year study of four hundred people exposed to the common cold. Results indicate that psychological factors influence the odds of infection. Some of these factors include a fighting spirit, social support, love and compassion, joy, optimism, hope, and mental relaxation.

Sandra M. Levy, an associate professor of psychiatry and medicine at the University of Pittsburgh School of Medicine, and colleagues found that the most important factor for a woman's survival from breast cancer was her level of joy. Women who considered themselves sad, hopeless, and worthless lived, on average, fewer than two years after the cancer's recurrence. Women with more positive attitudes lived much longer.

Although there are many psychological pitfalls and irrational beliefs that can contribute to pessimism, in truth, we are in control of our thoughts: We can be positive or negative, enthusiastic or dull, active or passive. Whether or not you stick to your detox diet and change your life is a matter of your choosing positive thinking and believing you are capable of creating a healthy life.

Test your thinking patterns by asking yourself these questions:

- Do I believe others cause my feelings?
- Am I always telling myself I "should" do this or that?
- Do I constantly criticize myself?
- Do I think I must do everything perfectly or not at all?

- Am I always apologizing for one thing or another?
- Do I feel as if I'm carrying the world on my shoulders?
- Is it hard for me to forgive and forget?
- Do I often feel helpless?
- Am I really hard on myself when I make mistakes?

If you've answered yes to many of these questions or if you frequently hear yourself saying or thinking "I can't," you consciously need to turn your thinking around *before* embarking on your detox plan. Believe in yourself, and realize that you are a capable person. Give yourself positive, encouraging statements. Don't feel as if succeeding with the detox program needed to be reinforced by others; if you do, you will feel helpless and out of control.

The first step in changing your attitude is to change your inner conversation. Make these statements to yourself:

- I am committed to completing the *Ten Day to Detox* program.
- I will keep my mind focused, set goals and priorities, develop a strategy for dealing with problems, and learn to relax.

- I will be courageous and change and improve each day. I will do my best and not look back.
- I will see change as an opportunity.
- I will keep track of my physical health and inner emotional life and be honest with myself.
- I will dream of success.

The Power of Prayer

For many, spiritual healing conjures up images of suspect TV evangelists. But that perception is fading as the effectiveness of prayer, not just by the patient but by another person, gains a measure of scientific respectability. In 1994 the National Institute of Health gave a thirty-nine-thousand-dollar grant to a researcher to study the role of prayer in curing drug and alcohol addiction, and several other studies investigating prayer are under way at universities across the country.

British scientists first attempted to measure the effectiveness of prayer on healing more than a century ago. But because medical journals showed little interest in the subject, much of the research appeared in obscure parapsychology publications, and most physicians did not know they even existed until recently. In his 1993 book *Healing Words,* Dr. Larry Dossey, who gave up his practice as an internist to write about spirituality and healing, reviewed more than 130 studies on prayer. He found that studies showed that prayer positively affected high blood pressure, asthma, heart attacks, headaches, and anxiety. Researchers, he noted, discovered that prayer also had an effect on the growth rates of bacteria, plants, fungi, and organisms. According to the studies, people who are compassionate can pray for themselves and others and achieve effects that are scientifically provable. Dossey added that it's not necessary to be religious or to believe in God, Goddess, Allah, Krishna, Brahma, the Tao, the Universal Mind, or the Almighty for prayer to work. One must only put his or her faith in the power of prayer.

As written in Romans 12:12, "Be constant in prayer." Prayer is a compelling method of preparation for detoxing. Ask for the strength to change, grow, cleanse, and be in control of your life. Pray to share your growth with others, to let you love those who support your endeavor as well as those who may try to put obstacles in your way. Fill your heart with forgiveness for your past indulgences, and encourage your spirit to work toward purification.

MOVING ON

Sit comfortably in a chair in a quiet place, with your feet flat on the floor and your hands in your lap. Close your eyes, and after a minute or so let your mind begin to say the word "open." When other thoughts intrude, ignore them and keep returning to "open." Don't think you have to repeat the word in a consistent way. Let it come and go and change speed. Make it the focus of your energy and attention, but don't force or concentrate too hard. It should come easily, as though you were hearing it rather than thinking it. Sit for around twenty minutes.

In the next chapter you will be taking a series of quizzes to help you discover your personal source of high-risk toxicity. Allow plenty of time to concentrate on this task.

> *Nobody sees a flower—really*
> *it is so small it takes time—*
> *we haven't time—and to see takes*
> *time.*
> *—Georgia O'Keeffe*

3

What's Your Personal Poison?

*The events in our lives happen in a
sequence in time, but in their
significance to ourselves, they find
their own order . . . the continuous
thread of revelation.*
—Eudora Welty

Each of us has a pretty clear idea of the kind of
person we believe we are: shy, adventurous, ten-
tative, perhaps weak or indecisive. It may well be
that this self-image is accurate, but the reasons
we travel our lives in the unique ways that we do
may not have as much to do with our personali-
ties as with our physical conditions. For example,
if you're feeling fatigued or nervous, headachy,
short-tempered, or anxious, you won't be open to
new experiences. Life's golden opportunities still

54

knock, but you're too depleted of precious energy to open the door. When loving relationships present themselves, you're likely to question your response, become suspicious, look for disagreements, fear intimacy.

Consider yourself a storage battery, directly, though invisibly, connected to the Big Source. As children we possess a strong connection. We have boundless energy, vibrating curiosity, original thinking, and open hearts. Our batteries are on "full charge." Our inner light glows. But as we grow older, the charge weakens, in part because of the toxic input previously discussed, everything from the foods we choose to eat and the air we breathe to the stress we create. It's not surprising that all this negative input blocks the healthy flow of energy.

THE SEVEN CENTERS OF ENERGY

According to ancient traditions, there are seven centers of energy within the body (chakras), corresponding to seven levels of consciousness and awareness. Think of the human body as a musical instrument having seven tones, seven different rates of vibration. Each tone has its unique place in music. If we are restricted to playing only one tone because our energy flow is blocked with toxins, we will produce a monotonous sound instead of a richly textured symphony. We will exist, but we will not really experience life. If we want to create beautiful, soothing music and have a spontaneous, creative, joyous, and abundant life, we must be able to move freely from note to note. Our bodies must be purged of the poisons that create unhealthy energy blocks and that prevent us from achieving the highest level of consciousness.

Gurudev Shree Chitrabhanu, a yoga master, illustrates the power of clear energy with this story:

There was a man in Bombay who became gravely ill. One day his son came to me and persuaded me to visit his father. When I saw the old man, he was too weak to move. It took two nurses to help him from his bed. Several days later, I read in the newspaper that a fire had broken out in the building in which he lived. This man was living on the seventh floor and there were no elevators, so I assumed that it would not have been possible to save him. Then, to my surprise, someone told me that this old man had been the first person to escape. While all the other tenants were gathering their belongings, he rushed ahead of them down the stairs. After a few days, I visited him especially to verify the story. Again I found him lying in bed with two nurses attending him.

"How did you climb down seven flights of stairs in your condition?" I asked him.

"I don't know," he said. "God sent me the energy."

Then I told him, "No, God did not send the energy. We always have that energy somewhere inside ourselves. Given the right conditions the energy can burst forth."

The old man's recovery was temporary and evoked by an emergency; his energy surged through, and he was able to make it to safety. Similarly, consider your life in a state of emergency. The fire may not be raging right outside your door, but your life's energy is burning away. How can you save it?

There's a lot of truth to the adages "Know thy enemy" and "Know thyself." Both ring true when it comes to change within ourselves. In this chapter you will learn to recognize your personal enemies, chip away at misconceptions, begin to see the light, to learn to "know thyself."

TAKING THE TESTS

After you complete the seven tests, tally your score, then study the analysis. I suggest you sit down in a quiet place, away from the television and radio, and preferably in a natural setting—either outdoors or by a sunny window—and work earnestly on this chapter. Tell yourself that you deserve uninterrupted time, and put yourself into this task wholeheartedly.

If you go deep enough with a "right" attitude, you will discover a bedrock of truth strong enough to create the foundation necessary for positive change.

SECTION ONE

PART I

Health Report

We often neglect to notice recurring ailments because we accept them as part of our natural constitutions. Complete this health report, keeping in mind that your original nature is wholeness, health. The following is a standard form used in many doctor's offices:

WHAT'S YOUR PERSONAL POISON?

Mark either *Never, Occasionally,* or *Frequently.*

General
— — — Allergy
— — — Chills
— — — Convulsions
— — — Dizziness
— — — Fainting
— — — Fatigue
— — — Fever
— — — Headache
— — — Loss of sleep
— — — Loss of weight
— — — Neuralgia
— — — Numbness
— — — Sweats
— — — Tremors

Muscle and Joint
— — — Arthritis
— — — Bursitis
— — — Foot trouble
— — — Low back pain
— — — Neck pain or stiffness
— — — Poor posture
— — — Swollen joints

Skin
— — — Boils
— — — Easy bruisability
— — — Dryness
— — — Hives
— — — Itching
— — — Rash

For Women Only
— — — Congested breasts
— — — Cramps
— — — Excessive menstrual flow
— — — Hot flashes
— — — Irregular cycle
— — — Painful menstruation

Habits
— — — Alcohol
— — — Coffee
— — — Drugs
— — — Tobacco

N O F   N O F

Gastrointestinal

— — — Belching or gas — — — Dental decay

— — — Colitis — — — Earache

— — — Colon trouble — — — Ear discharges

— — — Constipation — — — Ear noises

— — — Diarrhea — — — Enlarged glands

— — — Difficult — — — Eye pain

digestion — — — Gum trouble

— — — Excessive — — — Hay fever

hunger — — — Hoarseness

— — — Gallbladder — — — Sinus infection

trouble — — — Sore throat

— — — Hemorrhoids

— — — Nausea **Respiratory**

— — — Poor appetite — — — Chest pain

— — — Chronic cough

— — — Difficult

Eyes, Ears, breathing

Nose, Throat — — — Spitting up

— — — Asthma phlegm

— — — Colds — — — Wheezing

Total the number of *never* responses, *occasionally* responses, and *frequently* responses.

TOTAL/NEVER____

TOTAL/FREQUENTLY____

TOTAL/OCCASIONALLY____

Now take a few deep breaths and move on.

PART II

Diet

"Your food shall be your remedy." These words, written by Hippocrates more than two thousand years ago, hold true today as researchers continue to reinforce the connection between good nutrition and good emotional and physical health. Still, it's not only what we eat but also how, when, and why we eat what we do that is reflected in our well-being.

The following questions will bring to light those crucial dietary patterns.

1. When you spend the evening alone and boredom sets in, do you start to snack?

   —N   —O   —F

2. When planning meals, do you neglect to consider foods that are low in calories, fats, and additives?

   —N   —O   —F

3. During a coffee break do you resist the plate of fresh doughnuts that has been put out?

   —N   —O   —F

4. While cooking, do you find it nearly impossible to wait to eat until the meal has been prepared and end up munching while you chop and mix?

—N   —O   —F

5. Do you feel so virtuous when preparing a vegetable dish that you cook with butter, margarine, or other fats rather than use low-fat seasonings?

—N   —O   —F

6. When you experience disappointment or feel a little down, do you dig into that container of ice cream in your freezer?

—N   —O   —F

7. For convenience and taste, do you prefer to fry instead of grill, broil, or bake your food?

—N   —O   —F

8. Do you frequent fast-food restaurants?

—N   —O   —F

9. At fancier restaurants, when the dessert tray rolls around, are you likely to choose something gooey and rich rather than a bowl of fresh berries?

—N   —O   —F

10. When you're unhappy, rather than discuss your problems with a friend, do you seek the comfort of junk foods?

—N   —O   —F

11. Do you prefer to quench your thirst with an ice-cold soda rather than bottled water?

—N   —O   —F

12. Do you stop at the candy counter before going into the movie?

—N   —O   —F

13. You read about a "fad" diet that promises you can lose ten pounds in a week and still eat all the chocolate and chips you want.

—N   —O   —F

14. Do you eat fruit without washing or peeling the skin?

—N   —O   —F

15. Do you drink more than one cup of coffee (or tea) a day . . .

—N   —O   —F

16. . . . and put sugar and cream (or milk) in it?

—N   —O   —F

17. Do you buy foods without checking the labels for ingredients?

　—N　　　　　—O　　　　　—F

18. Do you tend to win the race when it comes to finishing your meals ahead of everyone else?

　—N　　　　　—O　　　　　—F

19. Do you skip meals because you are "too busy" and substitute filling snacks?

　—N　　　　　—O　　　　　—F

20. Do you drink alcohol?

　—N　　　　　—O　　　　　—F

21. Do you ever drink enough alcohol to give you unpleasant side effects of any kind?

　—N　　　　　—O　　　　　—F

22. When potato chips, salted nuts, and cocktail savories are around, do you find them impossible to resist?

　—N　　　　　—O　　　　　—F

23. Do you tend to dine out more than you eat at home?

　—N　　　　　—O　　　　　—F

24. Do you spread butter liberally on bread?
    —N   —O   —F

25. Do you avoid the food store that sells organic produce in your area because it's so expensive?
    —N   —O   —F

26. Do you consider whether produce is in season or grown locally?
    —N   —O   —F

27. Do you leave home without eating a vitamin-enriched breakfast?
    —N   —O   —F

28. Do you satisfy your sweet tooth whenever you have a craving?
    —N   —O   —F

29. Do you usually leave leftovers unrefrigerated because you know you're going to reheat them during the day?
    —N   —O   —F

30. When you order a hamburger, do you ask for it to be cooked either rare or medium-rare?
    —N   —O   —F

31. When you get to the shore, do you indulge in lobsters, clams, and oysters?

—N —O —F

32. Do you eat Chinese food without asking if it contains MSG?

—N —O —F

33. Will you buy chips with olestra so you can cut down on fat in your diet?

—N —O —F

34. Do you always seem to be on a diet?

—N —O —F

35. Do you pay attention to warnings about such additives as red dyes or sodium nitrite?

—N —O —F

36. Do you crave salty foods and liberally salt your dishes?

—N —O —F

TOTAL/NEVER____
TOTAL/FREQUENTLY____
TOTAL/OCCASIONALLY____

If you're feeling fatigued, this is a good time to take a small break. Will you go for a walk? Catch up on some work? Make a phone call? Lie down? Have a snack? Or ignore the break and just forge ahead? *Pay attention to your choice. Become conscious.*

> *Look and you will find it—what is*
> *unsought will go undetected.*
> —*Sophocles*

PART III

Your Environment

Often we're so busy carrying clouds of thought in our heads that we disregard our very surroundings. It's certainly happened to me. My husband might say, "Isn't that tree spectacular?" I'll give it a halfhearted look and then suddenly *really* see the tree bathed in a startling palette of autumn colors. Or I'll just happen to glance up at the night sky in winter while I'm bundled up from the cold and rushing from car to house. It's only then that my eyes feast on stars making trails like glittering tears and my soul is instantly nurtured. Bring the silver platter of awareness, I realize, and it will be laden with gifts.

On the other hand, sometimes the platter is so tarnished with toxins it can barely reflect the gifts. For example, when I've gone to meetings in New York City's big office buildings to talk with my editors, I feel full of energy while I take the elevator going up but drained and headachy on my way down. It must be the stress of the meeting, I think at first, forgetting to consider the other possibilities. Could it be new carpeting? Freshly painted walls? Stale air? Copier fluid? Fluorescent lighting? Or is it all that designer perfume?

By making you focus directly on your surroundings, this quiz will help determine how much the environment affects your well-being. Be as thoughtful as possible when answering the questions. If you've previously ignored the connection between your environment and your emotional and physical health, take this opportunity to stop and smell the formaldehyde.

1. Do you use products designed to kill household pests like ants, roaches, and fleas?

   —N   —O   —F

2. Do you use lawn or garden products that are chemically based?

   —N   —O   —F

3. Do you track these products into the house or neglect to wash your hands after using them?

 —N   —O   —F

4. Are there smokers in your home or at your place of employment?

 —N   —O   —F

5. Are you around a fireplace, wood stove, or kerosene heater?

 —N   —O   —F

6. How often do you run a vacuum cleaner?

 —N   —O   —F

7. Are your walls or ceilings damp from leaks or broken pipes?

 —N   —O   —F

8. Do you polish your furniture with commercial polishes or aerosol sprays?

 —N   —O   —F

9. Have you had wall-to-wall carpeting made from polyester or other man-made materials installed?

 —N   —O   —F

10. Do you use a humidifier, a dehumidifier, or an

air conditioner whose filter is not cleaned regularly?

　—N　　　　　—O　　　　　—F

11. Is your furniture covered with fabrics made from polyester, plastic, or other unnatural blends?

　—N　　　　　—O　　　　　—F

12. Is the copy machine in your office placed in an unventilated area?

　—N　　　　　—O　　　　　—F

13. Do you spend a lot of time in a city?

　—N　　　　　—O　　　　　—F

14. Do any windows in your home or office open onto the ground level of a city street?

　—N　　　　　—O　　　　　—F

15. Are the air-conditioned offices where you work separated by ceiling-to-floor partitions?

　—N　　　　　—O　　　　　—F

16. Do you use commercial cleaners in your home, especially those that contain ammonia or formaldehyde as their active ingredients (check the labels)?

　—N　　　　　—O　　　　　—F

17. Do you often avoid dusting (or do a half-hearted job), because it seems such a thankless chore?

   —N   —O   —F

18. Do you leave wet clothes lying around?

   —N   —O   —F

19. Do you have a water-damaged carpet that you just haven't gotten around to replacing?

   —N   —O   —F

20. Is your home painted with oil-based rather than water-based latex products? (Check labels on old cans for crystalline silica, ethylbenzene, or formaldehyde.)

   —N   —O   —F

21. Do your your shampoos, deodorants, and hair sprays contain aerosol propellants, ammonia, formaldehyde, or phenol?

   —N   —O   —F

22. Do you sleep on no-iron bed linens?

   —N   —O   —F

23. Do you have a number of clothing items that are permanent press or polyester-cotton fabric?

   —N   —O   —F

24. How often do you get your clothing professionally dry-cleaned?

—N   —O   —F

25. Do you bring your clothing home from the dry cleaner and hang it in the closet without first removing the plastic?

—N   —O   —F

26. Do you sit near a fax machine in your home or office?

—N   —O   —F

27. Do you keep your home at a relative humidity higher than 50 percent?

—N   —O   —F

28. Do you spray your house with indoor air fresheners or deodorizers?

—N   —O   —F

29. Have you purchased (or rented) a house without checking for radon? (Not applicable for apartment dwellers.)

—N   —O   —F

30. Do you keep an electric alarm clock right next to your bed?

—N   —O   —F

31. Are many of your teeth filled with mercury-based resins?

 —N   —O   —F

32. Have many of your teeth been bonded with sealants?

 —N   —O   —F

TOTAL/NEVER____
TOTAL/FREQUENTLY____
TOTAL/OCCASIONALLY____

Congratulations on the work you've done thus far. It's clear that you are serious in your desire to discover the influences that are affecting your health and limiting your potential. After taking these quizzes, you're probably more sensitive to environmental and dietary issues. Use this sensitivity to begin to clear out harmful toxins from your life. Later I'll go into greater detail and offer specific remedies.

Now is the perfect time to STOP! Return tomorrow to explore the relationship between toxic thought patterns and your physical being. The quizzes that follow in the second section will explore the emotional arena and require deeper contemplation.

*Learn to get in touch with the silence
within yourself and know that everything in
this life has a purpose.*
—Elisabeth Kübler-Ross

SECTION TWO

The Emotional Connection

Before responding to the questions in Section
Two, sit quietly on a straight-backed chair for five
minutes. When your mind is finally at peace, ask
yourself, "Who am I?" Become aware of the conflict between who you have been taught to think
you ought to be and who you really are.

Turn inward without judgment.

PART IV

Your Anger

1. When your feelings are hurt, do you need at
least a few hours (sometimes longer), before you
can talk about it?

   —N   —O   —F

2. How often do you feel disappointed or annoyed with your family and friends?

—N   —O   —F

3. Does your work at the office go unappreciated or unrecognized?

—N   —O   —F

4. Do you find it difficult to say what you're thinking if it isn't positive and upbeat?

—N   —O   —F

5. After a couple of drinks do you become silent, gloomy, or aggressive?

—N   —O   —F

6. Have you ever thrown things during a row with your spouse?

—N   —O   —F

7. Your partner or spouse nags you on a particular theme. Do you endure it but harbor resentment?

—N   —O   —F

8. When you have a hard day, do you take your annoyance out on the people closest to you?

—N   —O   —F

9. Last time you saw a movie you found highly offensive, rather than just walk out, did you complain to the theater manager, write a letter to a local newspaper, or protest in some other public way?

—N   —O   —F

10. You have been kept waiting half an hour at the doctor's office and you're on a tight schedule. Instead of complaining to the receptionist or calming yourself by browsing through magazines, do you just walk out?

—N   —O   —F

11. If a storekeeper is rude to you, do you display rudeness in return?

—N   —O   —F

12. A teenager drives by with rap music blaring from his stereo. Rather than remember the good old days when you used to drive around on high volume, do you feel your blood pressure start to rise?

—N   —O   —F

13. When very angry at an individual, do you hit or shove him or her?

—N   —O   —F

14. When stuck in traffic or behind a slow driver, do you quickly get annoyed?

—N —O —F

15. If someone criticizes you or treats you unfairly, are you likely to think about it for hours?

—N —O —F

16. When you read stories about the ravages of drugs in communities, do you think every drug pusher should be given the death penalty?

—N —O —F

17. If you're in line at the bank and someone at the teller's window seems to be inefficient, do you start to fume?

—N —O —F

18. When waiting for an elevator, do you press the button several times if the car doesn't immediately arrive?

—N —O —F

19. When someone is speaking to you, do your thoughts race ahead to what you want to say?

—N —O —F

20. If a friend has done something you morally

disapprove of, do you keep your feelings to yourself rather than discuss the issue right away?

  —N   —O   —F

21. If you get in a heated argument, can you feel
your heart pounding and your breath becoming
labored?

  —N   —O   —F

22. Someone bumps into you on a crowded street.
You know it's unintentional, do you still feel irritated?

  —N   —O   —F

23. Do you continue to feel resentment toward
your parents for the hurt they caused during your
childhood?

  —N   —O   —F

24. If someone is speaking very slowly during a
conversation, do you find yourself completing the
sentences?

  —N   —O   —F

25. Thanks to your strong opinions, you're the
one who chooses a restaurant or film. When the
choice is left to someone else, is it hard for you to
have a good time?

  —N   —O   —F

26. Are your moods pretty erratic?
    —N   —O   —F

27. When you are awakened in the middle of the night by loud music coming from your neighbor's apartment, do you go right over there and yell at them to "Be quiet!"?
    —N   —O   —F

28. Do you believe in *always* saying exactly what you think?
    —N   —O   —F

29. If your partner were unfaithful, would you blame the third party?
    —N   —O   —F

30. Do you find it hard to apologize?
    —N   —O   —F

TOTAL/NEVER____
TOTAL/FREQUENTLY____
TOTAL/OCCASIONALLY____

PART V

Your Level of Stress

1. On the whole, I'm not optimistic about my future.
   —N   —O   —F

2. Crowds make me feel a little edgy.
   —N   —O   —F

3. I always *have* to be on time.
   —N   —O   —F

4. I need to check things that I do several times before I'm satisfied.
   —N   —O   —F

5. I'm happiest when I'm kept really busy.
   —N   —O   —F

6. I often feel the need to cry but try to stifle the feeling.
   —N   —O   —F

7. I worry about past mistakes.
   —N   —O   —F

8. I know it's unreasonable, but still, I feel responsible for others' unhappiness.

    —N   —O   —F

9. I find it hard to relax.

    —N   —O   —F

10. I would describe my work as "pressured."

    —N   —O   —F

11. I'm bothered when things are out of order in my home.

    —N   —O   —F

12. I wake up unusually early because I feel I need to get a jump on the day.

    —N   —O   —F

13. I stay up late at night because either I'm having a tough time falling asleep or I want to get more accomplished.

    —N   —O   —F

14. I fantasize about running away.

    —N   —O   —F

15. Planning for a trip causes me more anxiety than excitement.

    —N   —O   —F

16. I tend to worry a lot.
    —N   —O   —F

17. If I'm fearful that I might create a problem, I won't say what I really mean.
    —N   —O   —F

18. I don't have a very lusty sex life.
    —N   —O   —F

19. I block out my feelings.
    —N   —O   —F

20. I'm a workaholic.
    —N   —O   —F

21. I will nap whenever possible to avoid unpleasant situations or feelings.
    —N   —O   —F

22. I talk fast.
    —N   —O   —F

23. There's a certain kind of family scene that I've come to dread.
    —N   —O   —F

24. It's my belief that some people (although not I) are born lucky.
    —N   —O   —F

25. Decisions over financial matters—bills, debts, taxes—weigh on me.

   —N   —O   —F

26. There is some material object that I feel I must have or my life won't be complete or satisfying.

   —N   —O   —F

27. If my "to do" list isn't completed at the end of the day, I'm upset.

   —N   —O   —F

28. My personal calendar is always packed.

   —N   —O   —F

29. I'm terrified of getting a debilitating or fatal illness.

   —N   —O   —F

30. Whenever I board an airplane, I seriously consider the possibility of a crash.

   —N   —O   —F

31. I find it difficult to do things if my usual way of doing them has to be altered.

   —N   —O   —F

32. Other than my spouse or lover, there's really no one with whom I can exchange confidences.

 —N   —O   —F

33. I think a pet would be just too much of a nuisance to keep.

 —N   —O   —F

34. I wish there were more than twenty-four hours in the day.

 —N   —O   —F

35. My relationship to the person closest to me is not truly a happy one.

 —N   —O   —F

36. I feel myself getting agitated and tense without good reason.

 —N   —O   —F

37. I find my life less pleasant than it might be because of noise created by aircraft, traffic, neighbors, etc.

 —N   —O   —F

38. I feel my success has been hindered by my background or upbringing.

 —N   —O   —F

39. I'm pretty unhappy with the way my body looks.

 —N   —O   —F

40. I regularly come in contact with people whom I actively dislike.

 —N   —O   —F

TOTAL/NEVER____
TOTAL/FREQUENTLY____
TOTAL/OCCASIONALLY____

PART VI

Jealousy, Insecurity, Envy

1. Your partner tries to speak to you about his sexual feelings and preferences. Do you respond by refusing to talk or trying to change the subject?

 —N   —O   —F

2. When your partner shows an interest in someone else, do you worry?

 —N   —O   —F

3. Do you believe that if the person who has

fallen in love with you discovers the *real* you, it will all be over?

—N —O —F

4. If you lost or damaged someone else's valued possession, would you avoid admitting you'd done it?

—N —O —F

5. You've gained ten pounds. Will you refuse to go out socially until you lose the extra weight?

—N —O —F

6. A friend accuses you of being selfish. Will you blame yourself and assume she must be right?

—N —O —F

7. If a friend recounted her vacation in great detail, would you respond by telling her all about the one you took last summer?

—N —O —F

8. When looking through the family photo album, are you likely to focus on the number of pictures there are of you, comparing yourself to other relatives?

—N —O —F

9. When your boss mistakenly compliments you

for a coworker's accomplishment, do you accept it without further explanation?

   —N   —O   —F

10. When your good friend forgets your anniversary, do you purposely let her birthday go by without uttering a word?

   —N   —O   —F

11. If your boss made unwanted sexual advances, would you suffer in silence?

   —N   —O   —F

12. You're asked to be maid of honor but to wear a dress that resembles a lampshade. Too embarrassed to wear it, do you politely decline the invitation?

   —N   —O   —F

13. You walk into a party where people are standing in groups, deep in animated conversations. Do you lean against the wall and wait for someone to come to you?

   —N   —O   —F

14. When talking to new acquaintances, do you find yourself comparing their clothes, figures, etc., to your own?

   —N   —O   —F

15. A former rival is moving back to town after ten years. Do you get your friends' support by bad-mouthing her before she arrives?

—N   —O   —F

16. Do you check your partner's pockets?

—N   —O   —F

17. If a colleague is promoted, are you likely to feel resentful that you weren't?

—N   —O   —F

18. If you were invited to a party that an old beau was attending with his new girlfriend, would you stay home?

—N   —O   —F

19. Someone is spreading nasty rumors about you. Would your first reaction be to go into hiding until the gossip dies down?

—N   —O   —F

20. When mistakes happen, do you think someone else has been careless?

—N   —O   —F

21. Do you go way over budget on an outfit that you're certain makes you look absolutely fabulous?

—N   —O   —F

22. When you compliment people, is your main concern whether they are grateful to you for the compliment?

 —N   —O   —F

23. Do you believe others don't appreciate your good qualities?

 —N   —O   —F

24. After arranging to take a day off from work to relax and enjoy yourself, do you worry about what your coworkers or boss are thinking about you?

 —N   —O   —F

25. Do you ever get the feeling that you are a "pretender"?

 —N   —O   —F

26. Do you believe that ultimately other people control your life, leaving you virtually powerless?

 —N   —O   —F

27. Do you spend more than an hour getting dressed before you're ready to go out for the day?

 —N   —O   —F

28. When a friend shares her good news—for ex-

ample, a promotion, new love, pregnancy—do
you feel jealous?

—N   —O   —F

29. Do you feel competitive with your friends?

—N   —O   —F

30. While at a party, you see your partner deep in
conversation with a very attractive person of the
opposite sex. Before your fear turns to fury, do
you head over to join them?

—N   —O   —F

31. Do you ever wish you were living someone
else's life?

—N   —O   —F

TOTAL/NEVER____
TOTAL/FREQUENTLY____
TOTAL/OCCASIONALLY____

> *We don't see things
> as they are,
> we see them
> as we are.*
> *—Anaïs Nin*

PART VII

Emotional History

As we grow up, our bodies become desensitized and our senses dulled as a means of self-protection; we "numb down" to prevent ourselves from feeling pain. Theories of child development vary greatly, but most share the view that in early childhood our attitudes toward ourselves and the world around us are formed through both positive and negative experiences. If our feelings become too difficult to bear, we erect defenses in order to survive emotionally. In the view of Wilhelm Reich and his followers, these defenses become imprinted in our bodies, creating muscle tension and blocking the energy that in health flows freely.

No scoring is provided for this section. Use its questionnaire as a tool to reflect upon your childhood and its impact on your present state of being. As you ponder the questions, you may experience a variety of unfamiliar body sensations or emotions because you are beginning to let go of feelings you have held on to for years, feelings of pain or pleasure, loneliness, sadness, joy, anger, or fear.

Sit with your feelings, and try not to chase them away. Keep in mind that you are on a journey of total cleansing. You need to unearth emotional toxins before you can make a commitment based on joy and inner peace.

Remember, *Only you are the wellspring of your life*.

1. Do you have memories before the age of three?
2. What is your earliest memory?
3. Is it painful to recall?
4. Are other memories pleasant?
5. Did your parents have a loving relationship?
6. Did you live in the same home when you were growing up, or did you move frequently?
7. Do you remember plenty of affection?
8. Were your parents divorced?
9. Where were you in the sibling chain?
10. Did you feel like a favored child, or do you believe that other siblings were more loved than you?
11. Did you suffer any severe illness in childhood?
12. Were you hospitalized?
13. Did you feel attractive as a child, or did you feel fat, homely, uncoordinated?
14. Were you popular in school?
15. Did you do well as a student?

16. Do you have any memories of your teacher or other children ridiculing you?
17. Were you sexually abused as a child?
18. Did you sexually abuse another child?
19. Were your parents supportive, or did they demean you?
20. Did you have a beloved role model outside the home?
21. Did you grow up in a religious home?
22. Did you attend a church or synagogue regularly?
23. If so, was this a pleasurable experience?
24. Was your family having financial difficulties when you were growing up?
25. Did your parents use spanking as a means of disciplining you?
26. Did your friends come to your house to play?
27. Did you have to "do without" material objects that other children possessed?
28. Did you envy them?
29. Did you steal as a child?
30. Were you a chronic liar?
31. Do you forgive yourself for digressions you might have committed during childhood?
32. Did you often harbor fantasies of running away?
33. Did you have a pet when you were growing up?

34. How old were you when you had your first consensual sexual experience?
35. Is it a pleasant memory?
36. Did you live with a stepparent?
37. If your parents were divorced, did they share joint custody?
38. What was your first experience with death?
39. Do you have memories of vacations shared with your family?
40. Are you close to your family now, including siblings?
41. If you are a parent, do you try to model your skills after your parents?
42. If the answer is no, why not?
43. Do you ever have dreams about the home in which you grew up?
44. Are they pleasant or anxious dreams?
45. Have you had any adult encounters with your family that were traumatic?
46. Or do you tend to let important issues slide?
47. On a scale of one to ten, how difficult was this questionnaire to complete?

The intensity or suddenness of your feelings may surprise you. If so, the questions may have revealed layers of feeling that have been suppressed and that up to now have been obstructed or hidden from your awareness.

Welcome these sensations; they are a sign that energy is moving. You are making deeper contact with yourself.

BEFORE MOVING ON

Congratulate yourself for completing the quiz section. Now total your test scores from all the quizzes.

	Never	Occasionally	Frequently
I HEALTH REPORT	____	____	____
II DIET	____	____	____
III YOUR ENVIRONMENT	____	____	____
IV ANGER	____	____	____
V STRESS LEVEL	____	____	____
VI JEALOUSY, INSECURITY, ENVY	____	____	____
TOTAL	____	____	____

If your highest score is in the *Never* category, your level of toxicity is lower than that of most Americans. You naturally gravitate toward a healthy diet and a clean environment. What's more, you've dealt with past traumas and for the most part, have let them go. Following the *Ten Days to Detox* program should not be particularly challenging for you. Scan your quiz results to focus on the areas that are most toxic for you, and keep them in mind during your fast.

If your score is highest in the middle range, *Occasionally,* you are like most of us, aware that you should eat a healthy diet and avoid stress and toxic situations, but until now have not made the committed effort. Here is your chance to take the reins and improve your life.

You may experience some unpleasantness at the start of the program as your body begins to detox. These effects should disappear by the third day of the program. Look over the quiz results to see which areas in your life are the most toxic. Make a conscious effort to eliminate them. Keep a journal to note the mental and physical changes you are experiencing.

You've scored most often in the *Frequently* column, and your level of toxicity is high. The detox program will be a challenge, but you will benefit most by its results. You're probably experiencing a number of effects from toxicity: fatigue, frequent colds, stomach discomfort and headaches, sleeplessness, insomnia, indecisiveness, depression, low libido, poor complexion, bloating, etc.

Let yourself imagine how different you will feel when you have completed the program.

I suggest that you take a sauna before starting the detox diet. When you sweat, you expel accessible toxins through your skin. Many spas and health clubs allow you to use their facilities on a daily rate. If not, soak in a warm tub, and follow up with a cold shower. Drink plenty of water while you're sweating. You might also consider arranging for a lymphatic drainage massage. (Chapter 5 familiarizes readers with other cleansing techniques.)

Do not be tempted to deviate from the program. Although the first few days may be difficult, you won't have to wait too long to start feeling the beneficial effects of the detox diet.

Get ready to change your life!

4

Ready, Set, Detox

*We are like the shining sun, and
our sicknesses, like passing clouds
which appear to extinguish the
sun's ray. The wise person who
gazes at the dull, gray sky knows
that, in reality, the sun still
shines brightly behind the veil of
clouds. All that is needed to uncover
its radiance is a clear, strong wind.*
—Buddhist teaching

A note of caution: The first rule of detox fasting is Fast only if you are feeling healthy and consult your doctor. Do not undertake a purification plan if you are suffering with flu or a chronic illness like diabetes and congestive heart failure, have an active ulcer or low blood pressure, are underweight, have an eating disorder, or are pregnant or breast-feeding. If you are taking any medications, be sure to check with your physician before embarking on the detox program. Many drugs behave differently on an empty stomach.

Also, don't fast during a period in your life when you have many physical or mental demands. All body cells—including those in the brain—rely on glucose as an energy source, and blood sugar level is maintained by the food we eat. When we are not taking in calories on a regular basis, blood sugar decreases, and our body systems may not work as effectively as during a nonfasting period. It's best to regard a fasting period as a time for reflection and rest, not as a time to go out and run a marathon or give an important presentation for your boss. In much the same way, holy fast days are usually linked to prayer and meditation.

The time of the month may even play a role in when a woman should choose to fast. Some studies indicate that the body has increased calorie demands after ovulation and before menstruation each month. It may be easier, then, to do without food in the beginning of the menstrual cycle than at the end. Some detoxing experts, like Dr. Elson Haas, the author of *Staying Healthy with the Seasons,* suggest that the two key times for natural cleansing are the times of transition into spring and autumn.

Most of us know that paying attention to circadian rhythms, the body's twenty-four-hour cycle—is critical to our well-being, but just as important is getting in sync with the seasons. Spring, for example, is a natural time to flush the toxins that have been building up all winter long. The layers of clothing we wear keep toxins trapped close to the skin, and cold air constricts our lungs, making deep, cleansing breaths nearly impossible. In fact, when we fight off a spring cold, it's our body's attempt to get rid of winter's toxic overload. According to Chinese medicine, the transition between the seasons is considered to be about ten days before and after the equinox or solstice.

My own experience tells me to consider a fast when I have the inspiration, the physical need, the spiritual desire, and the circumstances that will allow me to remain committed to the program. I would not suggest following the *Ten Days to Detox* program more than twice a year. However, I do recommend a twenty-four-hour fast each month, if you are healthy. Not only will your digestive system benefit, but you'll notice other changes: a two- to four-pound weight loss, a flat tummy, glowing skin, glossy hair, and energy to burn. During a daylong fast, consume at least eight six-ounce glasses of water, and keep physical activity to a minimum. When the need becomes apparent, I also do brief and modified three-day fasts. Samples of these fasts are included at the end of this chapter.

WHY A DETOXING FAST?

Fasting has long been a spiritual and physical means to purification. Both Moses and Jesus fasted for forty days; Luke denied himself food twice a week. Socrates and Plato fasted for ten-day stretches prior to beginning writing projects, Gandhi fasted as a form of political protest, and Hippocrates as a method of healing. Today Muslims fast annually during their holy period of Ramadan, and Jews on Yom Kippur, their Day of Atonement. Even animals fast. When ill, they instinctively know fasting will provide the rest and relaxation their body craves, helping it return to a more balanced and functional state. Fasting gives the digestive system, including the stomach, intestines, pancreas, gallbladder, and liver, a chance to minimize its activity. At the same time, abstaining from food increases the release of toxins from the colon, kidneys, bladder, lungs, sinuses, and skin.

As scientific studies show, fasting also boosts the immune system. At the University of Pittsburgh School of Medicine, researchers discovered an increase in the activity of infection-fighting white blood cells in a group of fasting obese volunteers. The same scientists also found that mice deprived of food for forty-eight to seventy-two hours had better resistance to a deadly microorganism than did well-fed animals. The Pittsburgh researchers theorize that fasting stimulates the release of chemical messengers known to spur the immune system.

Dr. Michael Pariza, of the University of Wisconsin, cites studies in which rats who had restricted food intakes had fewer instances of cancer and lived longer than rats on a regular diet. He suggests that steroidlike hormones produced in response to fasting may be able to repress cancerous cell growth.

Fasting has also been shown to improve the symptoms of rheumatoid arthritis. According to a study on twenty-seven patients in Norway, short-term fasting, followed by a vegetarian diet, produced a substantial reduction in disease activity. The study authors suggest that the improvement was due to changes in dietary fatty acids. Fasting is beneficial in the treatment of allergic and inflammatory conditions because it decreases the availability of arachidonic acid—a fatty acid found exclusively in animal products—which is converted in the body to compounds that promote inflammation. Many of the rheumatoid arthritis patients also benefited from another effect of fasting by eliminating allergy-inducing foods, such as corn, wheat, dairy, beef, and night-shades—eggplant and potatoes.

Fasting also encourages us to follow our true natures by clearing the path. During a detox program, self-realization and the desire for change are often stimulated; many people review aspects of their lives and end up questioning their relationships, jobs, and plans for the future. They are spiritually awakened, feel inspired, have greater mental and emotional clarity, sleep better, and are better able to make clear and useful decisions. While fasting, they can confront the core of problems that may have been buried for years. The feeling of liberation and the determination to eliminate obstacles and negative aspects of one's life are not unusual during abstention.

One of my friends, I'll call him Mark, was going through what he aptly coined his midlife freak-out. Suddenly his wife and family, whom he had always made his first priority, were feeling like heavy stones, burying him with responsibility and, he believed, destroying any chance of his real happiness. After a year of borderline depression he confided that he was thinking about ending the marriage. "It's not that I don't love my wife," he said, "but I'm just miserable."

I agreed Mark needed to get away, but I thought a fasting retreat would bring him the clarity he needed to see his life as a continuing journey possessing all the elements for joy. He just needed to "wipe the lens clean" so he could see anew and, in perfect perspective, appreciate all his blessings.

Mark, considering the alternative, agreed. He stayed in a bungalow (with kitchen) on the coast of Maine and, following my instructions, brought along all the food and water supplies he would need for his ten-day fast as well as a meditation cushion and a journal. He allowed himself plenty of walks along the beach and time to contemplate and write down his thoughts. He also strictly followed the fast.

On his return, Mark was a different man. His posture was erect, and his eyes were bright. He had an easy smile and was filled with positive, uplifting energy. Leave his wife? Mark wouldn't consider it. Instead he had plans for how their lives could only get better, and more important, he was grateful for the opportunity to "renew" and "re-create" his life.

Fasting not only helps you think about deeper issues but may also spark an exhilarating burst of energy. During a detox fast, the body increases its production of hormones so that it can facilitate the use of stored body fat in order to meet the increased energy requirement. One hormone is adrenaline, which can pump up feelings of vitality. Some people actually feel full of pep during a fast. Still, it is not the time to play three sets of tennis. Turn your energy inward.

MAKING TIME

Plan for your detoxing fast well in advance. Check off ten consecutive days on your calendar when you're unlikely to have to follow a hectic mental or physical schedule. It's ideal if you can set aside vacation time to fast. If not, be certain to make those close to you—family, friends, and co-workers—aware of your endeavor. Ask them to help out by sharing some of your usual responsibilities: Can your husband do the food shopping and cooking for the family? Can you hire a high school student to clean your house during the week, so that you won't feel compelled to run the vacuum? Will your boss allow you to forgo overtime for ten days? Can a neighbor, friend, or baby-sitter help shuttle the kids to various activities?

You can promise to repay favors generously. After completing the detox program, you will have energy and enthusiasm to spare. Activities that once seemed like drudgery will present themselves in a new light. You can also offer your services if your helpers express a desire to try the detox program. (After they see the results, I'm sure they'll be tempted.)

SETTING THE STAGE

In a perfect world you would begin your purification fast in a secluded cabin atop a mountain with startling vistas and a staff to attend to your every need—should you have any. Otherwise solitude and peace would be your companions.

But I'm a realist and have had to juggle my purification fasts with work and family. I'm confident that you can too. What you will need is a space all to yourself. Let the family know that you will be using the guest room, home office, laundry room, garage, or even bathroom as your safe haven when you need to be alone to relax, meditate, or write down your thoughts. At work, use your lunch hours as a time to retreat into yourself. Do not be tempted to join a colleague for lunch, even if you are planning just to sit across from her with a glass of water or a cup of tea. During this period in your life, choose to be alone as much as possible. Fellow fasters have reported closer feelings to their spiritual centers and desires to pray. If this happens, go with your desire. Be conscious of a new self emerging; allow yourself to be led by inspiration.

Also try to stay away from noisy, artificial environments. No trips to the department store, malls, or supermarket, if at all possible. Use this time to simplify your life. If the weather is accommodating, spend as much time as possible outdoors in the sunshine, taking leisurely walks and appreciating nature. Be sure to bring along your journal. Cold weather also has its allure, but you must dress warmly. Extra layers during detox are recommended since your body temperature may drop slightly during a fast.

The most important point to remember is that this is *your* time.

Leap into a new reality.

LET'S BEGIN

Most of us intuitively sense the benefits of a fast, but the idea of having to experience hunger is so unpleasant we try everything but a fast. Though vitamin and mineral products, herbal remedies, massage, sauna, meditation, and other practices are excellent complements to keeping your body in a healthy, pure state, their effectiveness is limited if your system, like those of most Americans, is toxically overloaded. There's just no way of getting around it: If you want to look and feel a decade younger, become revitalized and energized, give your digestive system a chance to relax, and boost your immune system, you need to follow a safe fasting program.

But a healthy detoxing fast does not mean that you just wake up one morning and stop eating. Getting the body ready for a fast is just as important as the fast itself, and the best way to prepare the body for fasting is by gently easing into it during the first three days of the program.

Preparation

During Days One and Two, prepare for your detoxing fast by reducing harmful influences from your diet. These include:

—Coffee and all caffeine products, such as chocolate, black teas, and colas*
—Alcohol
—Dairy products (milk, cheese, butter, ice cream, etc.)
—Eggs
—Sugar
—Refined and processed foods like white flour
—Meats
—Fried foods

* This limits the likelihood of suffering a caffeine-withdrawal headache, which can make abstention intolerable.

Read through the program. Shop in advance at a health food store for the items you will be eating during the next ten days, which include organic fruits, vegetables, whole grains, and herbal teas. These foods nourish and slowly detoxify the body so that actual fasting will be less intense. Also, be prepared to drink lots of liquids to prevent dehydration. And don't overdo it for the few days before you begin the program. Although many people view planned abstention as an excuse to splurge, experts advise the opposite tack.

"It's very important not to overeat the days before, but rather to consume light meals, high in complex carbohydrates and moderate in protein and fat," says Dr. George Blackburn, an associate professor at Harvard Medical School. "Feasting the day before a fast forces the body to handle metabolic extremes in terms of water and blood sugar levels and also heart rate. Besides stressing the body, this pattern of eating could actually make you more hungry than if you eat lightly."

Days One, Two, and Three

BREAKFAST
Upon awakening, drink eight ounces of spring water.

Then choose from one of the following:

½ CUP OATMEAL WITH RICE MILK

or

2 SLICES WHOLE GRAIN TOAST WITH 1 TEASPOON NATURAL PRESERVES (NO ADDED SUGAR)

or

FRESH FRUIT SALAD

HERB TEA (CHAMOMILE, PEPPERMINT, GINSENG)

—If you are used to sweetening your coffee or tea, use 1 teaspoon unprocessed honey or molasses.
—If you habitually drink more than 1 cup of coffee a day, switch to decaffeinated coffee for Days One and Two. Still, heavy coffee drinkers may experience some withdrawal symptoms. Regardless, *by Day Three you should be abstaining from all caffeinated products.*

LUNCH

1 BOWL VEGETABLE, LENTIL, LEGUME, OR CABBAGE SOUP WITH 3 WHOLE GRAIN CRACKERS

or

RAW VEGETABLE SALAD
3 WHOLE GRAIN CRACKERS

SNACKS

FRUIT, CARROTS, OR CELERY

or

1 GLASS FRUIT OR VEGETABLE JUICE

DINNER

WHOLE GRAIN PASTA WITH STEAMED VEGETABLES, PREFERABLY BEETROOT, CARROT, CELERY, CUCUMBER AND SPINACH

or

BROWN RICE WITH LEGUMES OR LENTILS

or

BAKED SQUASH OR POTATOES SPRINKLED WITH SESAME SEEDS OR TOPPED WITH A DOLLOP OF TAHINI

HERB TEA (no sweeteners)

Notes

—Drink at least six eight-ounce glasses of spring water throughout your ten-day detox.

—By Day Three all harmful foods should be completely eliminated from your diet.

—Whenever possible, prepare your meals with organic and whole grain foods.

—You will probably be experiencing some feelings of hunger. These will lessen as the program continues. Remember to eat slowly and chew your food carefully.

—Do not eat after 6:00 P.M.

—Take a sauna or hot bath. Brush your skin with a loofah or natural bath brush before you bathe to clear toxins from the skin. Do not use oils; they can clog pores and reduce the ability of your skin to "sweat" out toxins.

—Record your thoughts in your journal.

This is only the beginning of your great adventure. Savor the challenge.

Day Four

This is stage two of your detoxing program. You have already begun to give your digestive system a rest. During the next four days you will eliminate toxins from your body. Begin today with the Morning Brew, a juice that actively flushes toxins from your kidneys and liver.

BREAKFAST
Upon awakening, drink one eight-ounce glass of spring water.

Combine the Morning Brew:
1 CUP JUICE (PREFERABLY ORANGE IN THE WARMER MONTHS, APPLE OR GRAPE IN THE COOLER MONTHS)
1 TEASPOON VIRGIN OLIVE OIL
1 THIN SLICE FINELY CHOPPED GINGER

Blend until smooth and frothy.
Drink up!

1 CUP PEPPERMINT TEA

LUNCH
SMALL RAW VEGETABLE SALAD (1 CUP)

DINNER
SMALL FRUIT SALAD (1 CUP)

Notes
—Prepare a healing vegetable broth by using the *skins* of *organic* potatoes, carrots, and turnips, the outer leaves of cabbage, and slices of beet. Season with pepper and garlic. Do not use salt. You may sip this broth throughout the program *except* on Day Six, the day of abstention.

—*Drink six eight-ounce glasses of spring water* during the course of the day. The healing vegetable broth can be substituted for water.

—Sit quietly for ten minutes, and meditate. Concentrate on your breathing. Is it slowing down?

—Sensations of hunger will begin to subside. Are you feeling a sense of freedom? Clarity of thought? Deepening of reality? Write down your experiences in your journal.

Open to your new world.

Day Five

BREAKFAST
Upon awakening, drink one eight-ounce glass of spring water.

ADD 2 TEASPOONS OLIVE OIL TO THE MORNING BREW

1 CUP PEPPERMINT TEA

LUNCH
SMALL FRUIT SALAD

SNACK
VEGETABLE JUICE OF CARROTS, CELERY, BEETS, AND GREENS

or

HEALING VEGETABLE BROTH

Notes
—No food after 3:00 P.M.
—Don't forget to drink six eight-ounce glasses of spring water.

—Take a leisurely walk. Is nature speaking to you? Are you noticing details in your world that you once overlooked? Are you becoming more patient? Feeling at peace?

—To prepare for tomorrow, the Day of Abstention, try to go to bed early; aim for a full twelve hours of sleep.

When walking, just walk,
When sitting, just sit,
Above all, don't wobble.
                        —*Zen Master*

Day Six: Day of Abstention

By now your body is well on its way to cleansing and healing, ready for a full-day fast. This is my favorite day of the detox program, when I begin to appreciate fully the effects of the fast. The mind is alert; the body feels light and energized. This is an excellent time for walks in the country, meditating, journal writing, slow stretching, deep breathing, and soul-searching. Spend this day quietly with as much solitude as possible. Avoid the negative influence of those who do not understand or support your path.

Upon awakening drink *two* eight-ounce glasses of spring water.

ADD 3 TEASPOONS OLIVE OIL TO THE MORNING BREW

1 CUP PEPPERMINT TEA

Throughout the day drink plenty of water. It is necessary to *drink at least twelve eight-ounce glasses of spring water.*

Notes
- —If possible, arrange for a Reiki or polarity balancing session. Do not be tempted to have a vigorous massage during the Day of Abstention. Your body needs to be tended to in a gentle manner.
- —Luxuriate and turn your bathroom into a home spa. (There are recipes for homemade wraps and facials in Chapter 6.)
- —This is an excellent time to look through old photographs, letters, and diaries. Memories will be illuminated.
- —Meditate; breathe deeply; write in your journal.
- —Avoid stressful confrontations.
- —Listen to your inner voice. It is clear and spiritually attuned.

Look and you will find—
What is unsought will go
Undetected.
          —Sophocles

Day Seven

After the Day of Abstention the body is usually happy to continue without food. Regardless, follow the detox plan to health. This is not a test of endurance; it is a healthy program that leads to purification.

BREAKFAST
Upon awakening drink one eight-ounce glass of spring water.

ADD 2 TEASPOONS OLIVE OIL TO YOUR MORNING BREW

1½ CUPS NONCITRUS FRUIT SALAD (PREFERABLY MELON, PEACH, AND PEAR)

1 CUP PEPPERMINT TEA

SNACKS (up to 3)
VEGETABLE HEALING BROTH

or

GLASS FRESH-SQUEEZED VEGETABLE JUICE

Notes
  —Do not eat after 3:00 P.M.
  —Drink at least six eight-ounce glasses of spring water.
  —Remember to eat and drink slowly.
  —Separate yourself from the experience of everyday routines.
  —Your mind and body are now quiet enough to notice the small feelings that usually get drowned out. Cry! Laugh! Experience regrets! Applaud your accomplishments! Feel joy!
  —While you are still in a transitory state of fasting, continue to experience the greater mastery you have over your body.
  —Exercise gently. Stretches, slow walks, yoga, and tai chi are recommended. More strenuous exercise is suggested for tomorrow.

Embrace life!

Day Eight

The traditional way to break a fast in the Muslim religion is to eat a date and consume salt and water. This makes sense medically because the date contains potassium and other electrolytes that are easily lost during a fast, and the salt and water help build up blood volume again.

In the *Ten Days to Detox* program, you replace depleted glycogen stores by eating at least one small meal that is high in complex carbohydrates such as cereals, whole grain bread, pasta, or rice.

Don't be tempted to fall back into old patterns. You can do more harm than good by haphazardly breaking a purification fast.

BREAKFAST
Drink one eight-ounce glass of spring water upon awakening.

ADD ONLY 1 TEASPOON OLIVE OIL TO YOUR MORNING BREW

1 SMALL BOWL OATMEAL WITH RICE MILK

or

1 SMALL BOWL GRANOLA WITH RICE MILK

1 CUP PEPPERMINT, GINSENG, OR CHAMOMILE TEA

LUNCH
1 SMALL RAW VEGETABLE SALAD WITH MISO DRESSING

1 SLICE WHOLE GRAIN BREAD SPREAD WITH PEANUT, CASHEW, OR TAHINI BUTTER (optional)

or

ASSORTED FRUIT SALAD WITH SUNFLOWER SEEDS

3 WHOLE GRAIN CRACKERS

SNACK

1 CUP HEALING VEGETABLE BROTH

or

NONCITRUS FRUIT

or

FRESH VEGETABLE JUICE

DINNER

WHOLE GRAIN PASTA or RICE WITH STEAMED VEGETA-BLES

or

SWEET SQUASH or 2 BAKED POTATOES SPRINKLED WITH SESAME SEEDS

1 CUP OF GREEN LEAFY VEGETABLES

or

BROWN RICE WITH LEGUMES OR LENTILS

Notes

—Your digestion has been at rest, so you need to go slowly and chew your foods very well.

—Stick to small portions; do not overeat or make any meal substitutions.

—Coming back into foods is a crucial time for learning. Keep notes. What foods have you been desiring? What has your sleep pattern been like? Has your energy level increased?

—Try a session of mirror gazing. Does it feel

much different from before the fast? Many fasters report feeling self-love rather than self-loathing during a detox. Is this your experience?

—While you're cleansing out your body, why not rid your home of toxins as well? Look to Chapter 6 for guidelines.

—Increase your exercise. Take a longer walk; go for a leisurely swim; you might opt for a short, nontaxing bicycle ride. No vigorous aerobic exercise.

Days Nine and Ten: Reentry

Good news: No more Morning Brew!

BREAKFAST
Drink one eight-ounce glass of spring water upon awakening.

1 BOWL OATMEAL WITH RICE MILK

or

1 BOWL GRANOLA WITH RICE MILK

or

2 SLICES WHOLE GRAIN TOAST WITH NATURAL PRE-SERVES

1 SMALL FRUIT SALAD OR FRESH-SQUEEZED FRUIT JUICE

1 CUP PEPPERMINT, CHAMOMILE, GINSENG, OR GINGER
TEA

or

OTHER HERB TEAS OF YOUR CHOICE

LUNCH
1 SMALL BOWL STEAMED VEGETABLES WITH TOFU ON A
BED OF RICE

or

RAW VEGETABLE SALAD (ADD AVOCADO)

SNACK
3 WHOLE GRAIN CRACKERS WITH ORGANIC PEANUT BUT-
   TER

or

1 SMALL BOWL HEALING BROTH

or

FRESH FRUIT (NONCITRUS)

DINNER
WHOLE GRAIN PASTA WITH STIR-FRIED VEGETABLES (USE
OLIVE OIL)

or

BAKED BUTTERNUT SQUASH AND POTATO PLATE

or

BROWN RICE AND LEGUMES OR LENTILS

DESSERT (OPTIONAL)

FRUIT SMOOTHIE

BLEND 2 CUPS FROZEN FRUIT WITH 1 CUP WATER UNTIL SMOOTH

Your *Ten Days to Detox* fast is over, but your lifelong journey has just begun. Below I offer short-range fasts with long-lasting results. Now that you've experienced the pleasure of a detoxing fast, you might think about making it a regular part of your life.

In the following chapter you'll read about the detoxing effect of exercise, as well as breathing, massage, and meditation techniques. Next you'll learn about how you can clean up environmental toxins from your home and office and how you can turn your bathroom into a cleansing home spa.

But before you move on, stop. Sit quietly for ten minutes. Follow your breath.

> *Visualize a river.*
> *Quietly watch the*
> *beautiful, flowing water*
> *and see yourself*
> *and your life*
> *finally floating*
> *smoothly.*

ONE DAY TO DETOX

I've found that fasting once a week helps me focus mentally and physically. Usually I choose Sunday when the family naturally slows down and there are fewer demands made. Frankly I look forward to my fasts, especially if I've had an especially stressful week.

The primary function of the shortened fast is to allow the organs of the body to rest and go through a general, quick-fix housekeeping. You won't be "scrubbed clean" the way you are after the ten-day detox, but you'll definitely feel a difference. This fast will facilitate the excretion of organic and inorganic poisonous substances, such as iodine, arsenic, and mercury, as well as acids, viral agents, and oxalates. These are tough for the body to eliminate under ordinary circumstances. Their expulsion is greatly facilitated during a fast since the activity of many internal organs is altered.

The carbohydrates, proteins, fats, vitamins, minerals, trace elements, and water we ingest are modified by the internal organs through a complex series of metabolic reactions before they can be used by the body. But the majority of these reactions, such as intestinal digestion, nutrient transport, and excretion via the lungs and skin, continue even when we are not eating. The liver alone can store proteins and up to a seventy-two-hour supply of glycogen (stored carbohydrates), which can offer cells nutrients for growth and maintenance. Typically, after energy and protein reserves have been depleted, the body may break down cells to provide the missing nutrients in a process called autolysis. Fat will be broken down, thereby reducing stored body fat levels. Protein requirements will be met first with proteins found in the bloodstream and later from the breakdown of inferior tissues, such as old, damaged, or abnormal cells.

Even though you're fasting for only twenty-four hours, your stomach and intestines will probably shrink a bit. The excretion of digestive juices will decrease, and your intestines will change from being organs of absorption to organs of excretion. The excretion of waste products and toxins will also take place in the liver and other organs participating in the digestive system. Clearly a once-a-week detoxing program offers continuous as well as a few dramatic results. Try it for a month.

THE WEEKLY TWENTY-FOUR-HOUR FAST

Drink between eight to twelve glasses of fresh spring water throughout the day.

BREAKFAST
1 LARGE GLASS FRESHLY SQUEEZED ORANGE OR GRAPE-
FRUIT JUICE (OR 1/2 LEMON SQUEEZED INTO 1 GLASS
SPRING WATER)

MIDMORNING SNACK
1 CUP HERBAL TEA WITH A SMALL AMOUNT OF HONEY,
IF DESIRED

LUNCH
1 LARGE GLASS FRESHLY EXTRACTED VEGETABLE JUICE

DINNER
1 LARGE GLASS FRESH VEGETABLE JUICE

LATE SNACK (if desired)
1 CUP HERB TEA

THE THREE-DAY JUICE FAST

I recommend this fast as a way to start the first
week of each new season *only* when you're not
planning to celebrate the change of season with a
ten-day detox. This is a particularly strenuous
detox diet that requires commitment and a slowing down of activity.

Drink between eight and twelve glasses of fresh spring water each day of the three-day fast.

FLUSH

1/2 CUP FRESH ORANGE
   OR LEMON JUICE (warm months)
   OR APPLE JUICE (cooler months) (use fresh-squeezed or pressed organic juices)

1 THIN STRIP GINGER, CHOPPED

2 CLOVES GARLIC, CHOPPED

8 OUNCES OF NATURAL SPRING WATER

Drink 2 glasses of mixture—one in the A.M.; one before 3:00 P.M.

MIDDAY SNACK

8-OUNCE GLASS FRESHLY SQUEEZED VEGETABLE JUICE

You may also drink unlimited amounts of water, peppermint, and chamomile teas.

Raw juice fasts in general are rich in enzymes (organic catalysts), which increase the rate at which foods are broken down and absorbed by the body), thus enabling an immune system that is healing or recovering to absorb more comprehensively the valuable nutrients it needs.

Many valuable enzymes found in fruits and vegetables are destroyed when they are cooked or processed. That is why fresh raw produce should constitute 50 percent of a detoxing diet. A diet that is 50 to 75 percent raw can increase energy by 50 percent, according to the Hippocratic Health Institute, and help retard and even reverse the degenerative process. Juice fasting (even short term) supports the immune system through a wide variety of healing processes from allergies to viral herpes. During a fast, the tissues, membranes, and bloodstream all are cleansed of toxins.

As in all fasts, break this one slowly by introducing small portions of clear soups, steamed vegetables, and different fruit juices. Remember to chew slowly and savor the introduction of new tastes.

5

Purifying Body and Spirit

No doubt after completing your *Ten Days to Detox* program, you feel completely renewed. Your senses are alive, perceptions powerful; your body feels lithe and strong. When you look in the mirror, you are astounded to see a bright-eyed, youthful reflection returning your gaze. Acquaintances may have remarked about the change. They may have asked, "What's different about you?" wondering whether you've just returned from an expensive spa or perhaps had some plastic surgery; good friends will generously compliment you on your appearance. It will be clear to you and those around you that you have changed.

You can easily pat yourself on the back now and return to your old ways. But if you do, it won't take long to fill your body and emotional life with toxins once again. All your hard work will be like a passing cloud. What a terrible waste of energy!

My Zen teacher once asked us, "If you were looking for water, would you drill fifty holes of one-foot depth or one hole that was fifty feet deep?" In each case the effort is the same, but the results are different. We can choose to dissipate our energies, thinking we can return to our lives and just occasionally dig a foot here or there to cleanse ourselves, or we can make a commitment, concentrate our attention, time, and muscle on digging in the direction of pure health until we tap it. Once done, we can forever enjoy the wellsprings of our lives.

The good news is that you've already accomplished the most difficult part of a detoxing program. You've begun. The rest is a piece of cake (carrot, of course!).

The techniques described in this chapter will help you maintain the purified state you have worked so hard to attain. Choose those methods that fit into your lifestyle and feel "right" for you. Don't worry about the time commitment; we all have such hectic lives. Many of these methods require only a few minutes out of your day, others an hour or two a week.

For my personal program, I've chosen to meditate twenty minutes daily; I "sit" in the morning when my body is rested and full of energy and my mind is not yet engaged in the activities of the day. I also have a sauna every other day, alternately with my home spa hour, and exercise aerobically four times a week. Once a week I fast on fruit juices and herb teas. Twice a year, at the start of autumn and spring, I take advantage of the ten-day detox program. For a diet I avoid fried or processed foods as well as dairy products, and I eat plenty of organically grown fruits and vegetables and whole grains. On special occasions, when gift giving is in order, I request a massage certificate from friends and loved ones.

Most important, I try to surround myself with positive and loving energy. If a relationship "feels" bad, I've learned to trust that feeling. I've burned a lot of bridges in my lifetime and rarely regretted it. There's no reason to allow negative feelings and unpleasant situations to intrude on your inner peace.

If you're committed to keeping your body and spirit clean, it's a good idea to first read this chapter completely. Consider the techniques that seem appealing to you. Next, write out a program that you think is compatible with your lifestyle.

After you've tried your chosen methods, if something doesn't feel right, substitute one technique for another. All the options described will help you maintain a purified state.

DETOX BREATHING

> *The regulation of the breath brings*
> *all happiness material and*
> *spiritual from the acquisition of*
> *Kingdoms to Supreme Bliss.*
> *Therefore, Oh! Rama! Study the*
> *Science of the Breath.*
> —*Sage Vasishta*

Breathing is a crucial way to detox our emotional and physical bodies. But because it's involuntary, most of us take it for granted, and we do it all wrong. In one year an average adult with bad breathing habits inhales about four to five tons of oxygen, but only a thousand pounds of it are actually used; we get only *half* the oxygen we need and expel only half the carbon dioxide we should. We end up robbing our lives of energy and leaving our cells clogged with toxins.

This high level of carbon dioxide in the blood causes the body's flight or fight mechanism to kick in and the carotid artery, the main artery to the brain, to constrict. The result is a buildup of harmful stress that surges through the body, attacking the immune system.

Studies have shown that stress can send emergency hormones flowing into the bloodstream and may help cause brittle bones in women, infections, and even cancer. "In extreme cases, this hormonal state destroys appetite, cripples the immune system, shuts down processes that repair tissue, blocks sleep and even breaks down bone," reports Dr. Philip Gold of the National Institute of Mental Health.

"Overbreathing can amplify ordinary tension to a harmful degree," adds Herbert Fensterheim, a New York psychologist who teaches his patients to retrain their breathing. "On the other hand, when we breathe freely, the diaphragm, belly, and chest undulate with the rhythm of each breath, and the whole body is energized with life-giving oxygen." Fensterheim suggests watching a young child or an animal breathe and observing how the body moves when the breathing is natural and relaxed. "As adults most of us have lost this knack. We breathe shallowly," says Fensterheim. "We just don't make full use of our diaphragms."

Muscular tension, tension that has evolved over years of poor posture, is largely to blame for our shallow breathing. But we may also unconsciously restrict our breathing as a way of suppressing painful emotions, for the depth of our breathing is also related to the richness and intensity of our feelings. Many of us have learned to control rather than to express our deepest feelings, and this inevitably means tightening our breathing muscles and tensing our chests or bellies, the seat of our feelings. In the process of distancing ourselves from feelings of sadness, anger, or fear, we also block the free flow of purifying energy in the body and diminish our capacity for pleasure.

During Zen meditations our teacher implored us to "Breathe down! Squeeze your kidneys! Purify!" After years of practice I could actually feel my breath sinking down, lingering in my kidneys. At these moments my meditations were more satisfying; thoughts flew away like so many restless sparrows. Sitting time passed quickly, and I felt ineffable joy radiating from my kidneys to my navel and up to the so-called third eye.

On a more grounded note, menopausal women who want to reduce their intake of estrogen may find the answer by changing their breathing patterns. A study at Wayne State University School of Medicine in Detroit concluded that shallow breathing may contribute to menopausal hot flashes and that slow, deep breathing helps reduce their frequency.

In order to change your breathing habits, it's a

good idea first to become aware of them. Monitor your breathing while you go about your daily life. From time to time just observe your breath. You will begin to see that thoughts or feelings can disrupt your natural rhythm and make you hold back your breath.

The following exercises will help you relax and cleanse your system. With practice you'll be able to change your negative breathing patterns, gain vitality, and achieve a calmer state of mind and a cleaner, healthier body.

• For full breathing, lie on the floor, resting your hands on the sides of your rib cage just above the waist, and exhale completely. Inhale slowly through the nose, letting your abdomen rise as much as possible, for five seconds; continue breathing in for another five seconds, expanding and filling your rib cage. Hold for five seconds. Now slowly exhale through the mouth for ten seconds, expelling all the air from your chest down to your abdomen.

• Lie on your back with your upper body propped up on a pillow at about a thirty-degree angle. Place a telephone book on your stomach to make sure you're breathing with your abdomen, not your chest. Focus your attention on your nostrils, and gently inhale, concentrating on the feeling of taking air in through your nose. Next, gently exhale, and completely relax one group of muscles (shoulders, arms, legs), letting them go limp and heavy. Once you've exhaled fully, breathe in again, continue the process, and switch muscle groups for eight to ten minutes. Try this exercise once a day.

• While sitting in a straight-back chair, block one nostril with the thumb and the other with the third finger. Using the ratio 1:4:2, inhale through one nostril, hold the breath, and exhale through the other nostril. For example, using this ratio, breathe in through your right nostril to the count of four, retain the breath for sixteen counts, and exhale through the left nostril, counting eight. Wait approximately fifteen seconds, and repeat the exercise, now inhaling through the left nostril and exhaling through the right. According to your capacity, you may increase the number of counts you breathe and retain the breath on the basis of the same ratio. Complete this exercise five times. (This is an excellent technique for taking oxygen deep into the lungs and all the blood cells and for releasing the carbon dioxide from the body. It's also useful for calming and focusing the mind.)

• Wayne State University Professor Robert Freedman's method for reducing hot flashes: The goal is to cut your breathing rate in half.

Instead of taking fourteen to sixteen breaths per minute, take six to eight. You can use slow breathing as a preventive measure or as an on-the-spot treatment once you feel a flash coming on. Practice it twice a day for fifteen minutes each time for preventative purposes. If you feel a flash beginning to hit during a stressful or warm situation, start slowing down your breathing immediately.

MASSAGE

> *Here in this body are the sacred*
> *rivers: here are the sun and moon*
> *as well as all the pilgrimage*
> *places. . . . I have not encountered*
> *another temple as blissful as my*
> *own body.*
>
> —*Saraha*

In the last decade massage has enjoyed a surge of popularity. Once thought of as a luxury for the pampered, it has become a favorite of stressed-out office workers, recreational athletes, and those of us who appreciate its ability to cleanse and relax both our bodies and our minds.

Massage's benefits go way back; it's an ancient healing art mentioned in Chinese literature as early as 3000 B.C., and Greek and Roman physicians used it to treat their rulers. "Massage has its roots in earliest medicine," says Richard van Why, president of the Texas-based Bodywork Research Institute. "It's always been a crucial part of the health systems of most cultures."

Research shows that massage boosts circulation to the skin's surface, bringing along a greater supply of nutrients and encouraging self-cleansing. By increasing the blood flow, massage also hastens the removal of metabolic waste products from the body. It fuels the muscles with fresh oxygen, releases physical tension, and soothes the nerves. The result is a blend of cleansing, relaxation, rekindled energy, and healing.

"Across all the medical studies on massage," says Tiffany Field, a professor of pediatrics, psychology, and psychiatry at the University of Miami School of Medicine and the director of its Touch Research Institute, "we see a decrease in anxiety and depression, an improvement in sleep and a reduction of stress hormones such as cortisol and epinephrine."

Field also contends that kneading the muscles stimulates the vagus nerve, the largest and most complex of the cranial nerves that link the brain to the heart, and that it can affect speech, alertness, and relaxation as well as release stress hormones. "Touch," she says, "affects digestion and the release of hormones like insulin, which promotes the absorption of food and might help explain why premature infants who are massaged gain weight."

In a three-month test nineteen asthmatics who received weekly fifteen-minute upper-body massages reported drops in chest tightness, wheezing, physical pain, and fatigue. The study was presented at the American Academy of Allergy, Asthma and Immunology.

Thomas J. Birk, director of the Morse Research Center at the Medical College of Ohio in Toledo, has tied the art of touch to the science of molecules and medicine in a controlled study of people infected with HIV. Before and after massage, blood tests measured the number of natural killer (NK) cells, which form part of the immune system. "Everyone who got massages felt better during the twelve-week period," Birk says. "More important, their cell counts improved."

Douglas DeGood, a researcher at the University of Virginia, demonstrated that as part of post-surgical care for women undergoing hysterectomy, a daily forty-five-minute massage reduced stress hormones, significantly lowered blood pressure, and aided the healing process. In his study the women receiving massage required no posthospitalization physician care in the four-week follow-up period, whereas a third of the women in the control group needed doctor visits.

In order to keep your body cleansed and relaxed and to boost your immune system, I recommend at least a bimonthly massage. Your health insurance will most likely cover massage therapy if your doctor prescribes a specific number of sessions and precisely states the desired outcome. Orthopedists, neurologists, and internists are the doctors most likely to recommend massage to their patients.

Most Common Methods of Massage

SWEDISH (WESTERN STYLE)

This type of massage is an all-purpose method to get the blood moving and promote general well-being. Featuring long, gliding strokes, Swedish massage is oriented to physiology, specifically dealing with blood flow and contracted muscles.

SHIATSU

This form of acupressure and massage has a spiritual goal to get the mind and body in harmony. Used widely in Japan for more than one thousand years, shiatsu is derived from traditional Chinese medicine. It postulates that chi, or life energy, flows along invisible body pathways called meridians. Poisons build up and illness occurs when energy becomes blocked at specific pressure points.

REFLEXOLOGY

Practitioners of this method of massage say that the feet are the mirror of the body and that various reflex areas in the feet correspond to parts of the body. Each of the seventy-two hundred nerve endings in the foot is connected via the spinal cord and brain to specific organs and glands like a map. Your toes (which correspond to your head) lie north, and your heels (which correspond to your intestines) lie south. Reflexologists apply pressure to these spots on the feet and hands to promote the health of the corresponding body part, organ, or gland. The most immediate benefit is a general sense of well-being and relaxation, but Manhattan-based reflexologist Laura Norman, author of *Feet First,* says that "during a cleanse, you can use reflexology to speed elimination, and energize and ease detox side effects like headache and nausea."

CRANIOSACRAL

This type of massage uses the ultimate form of soft touch—holding and cradling—to coax the bones of the cranium (skull and face) and the sacrum (pelvis) to release tension and to promote the flow of cerebrospinal fluid. It's a combination of subtle manipulation, energy work, and realignment.

LYMPHATIC DRAINAGE

My personal choice, lymphatic drainage massage, kneads deep muscle tissue and reduces the accumulation of toxic fluids by targeting superficial lymph tissue. Lately the buzz has been that it can also banish cellulite. The theory: Lymphatic drainage breaks up fluid buildup, smoothing out the dimply texture of skin. "If there is fluid in superficial tissues, lymphatic drainage may help reduce the appearance of cellulite," says Joachim Zuther, director of the Academy of Lymphatic Studies in Miami, Florida, "but the technique was designed as a detoxing method, not as a superficial beautifier."

Finding a Therapist

Massage therapists at local Ys, health clubs, salons, or day spas are usually screened by the American Massage Therapy Association, but it's still important to ask for credentials (some states license massage therapists). Inquire whether the therapist belongs to a professional association or has received at least five hundred hours of training at an accredited school. Word of mouth is another good way to find a massage professional, especially a freelance therapist who will come to your home.

Self-Massage

If you don't have the finances to cover bi-monthly massages, or you want to increase their frequency without breaking your bank account, self-massage is a satisfying alternative.

• This requires the proper setting. Warmth, comfort, quiet, and low light are all essential. Find a position that is relaxing and comfortable. Lying on your back or side may be good for some parts, but for others it's easier to sit or kneel down. Have a fragrant body lotion or massage oil ready for use if you need it. Work slowly and rhythmically, closing your eyes so that you can focus all your attention on sensation. You need have no set routine, but I found the following technique to be most effective:

• Begin by exploring your face thoroughly, as if you were a blind person learning to recognize it for the first time. Work more deeply with your thumbs and fingers around any areas of tension, like the jaw muscles or eye sockets.

• Repeatedly comb your fingers through your hair, or gently rub your scalp, as if you were shampooing. Place your hands, fingers spread apart, on top of your head. Press down, and rub your scalp in a small, circular motion. Move your fingers a half inch closer to your forehead, and repeat. Continue massaging until you reach your hairline; place the index fingers on the temples, and massage the area. This massage is immensely relaxing and effective in relieving toxic tension, especially if you're the kind of person, like me, who tends to live in her head.

• If you spend a lot of time in front of a computer, your shoulders and neck are probably tight and knotted. Massage both shoulders at once, or do first one side with your opposite hand, then the other side. Starting at the base of your neck, massage along your shoulder until you reach the top of your arm. Press fingertips deeply into the back of your shoulder as you massage.

• Exploring one of your own hands with the other is an unusual sensation at first, since we're used to shaking or holding hands with others. But it gives us the unique opportunity to see how it feels to give and receive at the same time. Try working your thumb into the fleshy areas of the palm and stretching and squeezing each finger.

• We often neglect our feet, forgetting the service they do us every day. Yet massaging your own feet can be immensely beneficial and relaxing. Try working across the sole with your fingers or thumb or stretching and pulling the toes.

• You can also experience self–lymphatic drainage massage. Here's how: Beginning under your ears and using both hands, stroke down your neck and throat to the hollow above your collarbone. Do this about fifteen times. Now cross your arms over your chest. Press your index and middle fingers into the hollow above your collarbone, and circle in opposite directions. Repeat fifteen times. Next, raise one arm and massage your armpit in circles ten times. Repeat on the other side.

• Complete your massage by lying down and totally relaxing for twenty minutes.

On-the-Job Massage

Whenever you've got to muster courage—to talk to your boss, for example, or make a presentation—take a few minutes to do this simple massage technique: With the fingertips of both hands, gently touch the skin above each eye, midway between your hairline and your eyebrow. Massage in a small, circular motion for three to ten minutes while imagining everything's going your way. This massage increases blood to the brain, which will help you think creatively and work at your top potential.

NOTE: Although most people find massage an effective, safe treatment for a host of illnesses, medical experts warn anyone with a history of blood clots, diabetes, a recent fracture or sprain, or a high fever to avoid it. Doctors also recommend caution to those with circulatory, skin, or cardiac problems. If you have a chronic health problem, consult your doctor for advice.

SAUNA

All over America, people are perspiring freely.
—Mademoiselle
(July 1993)

An old Finnish saying describes the sauna as "a sacred place, a place of silence, a place of recreation, a place of peace, and a place of health." In medieval times healers relied on saunas to cure illnesses, and priests used their heat to chase away evil spirits. Today the sauna is an integral strategy in the purification program, and I personally couldn't get by without taking a sauna at least three times a week. A sauna eliminates toxins, including sodium, alcohol, and nicotine, and potentially carcinogenic heavy metals, like cadmium, lead, and nickel. These toxins, accumulated in the system through sluggish elimination, are normally removed from the body by perspiration. The sauna increases the eliminative, detoxifying, and cleansing capacity of the skin by stimulating the sweat glands.

While we perspire in a sauna, the metabolic processes of our vital organs are increased and the growth of pathogenic bacteria and viruses is slowed down. A sauna creates a "fever" reaction that kills potentially dangerous viruses and bacteria and increases the number of leukocytes in the blood, thereby strengthening the immune system. If you sauna regularly when a flu epidemic hits your area, you should be able to avoid infection.

The sauna also provides the body with a cardiovascular workout. While in the sauna the body absorbs considerable heat, and since the natural reaction is to cool down, blood is diverted away from the inner organs to the extremities and skin. This involves substantial increases in heart rate, cardiac output, and metabolic rate. Ultimately taking a sauna is a very effective cardiovascular exercise that, when experienced regularly, increases aerobic fitness.

You'll also lose weight, and not just from water loss; water doesn't "leak out" of the body. Instead sweating is part of the complex thermoregulatory process of the body involving substantial increases in the heart rate, which use up considerable energy. A moderately conditioned person can easily "sweat off" a pound in a sauna, consuming nearly three hundred calories; a heat-conditioned person can sweat off six to eight hundred calories. (An average person burns off three hundred calories during a three-mile run.) Therefore, while the weight of the water loss can be regained by rehydration, the calories consumed will not be.

What's more, saunas stimulate the vasodilation of peripheral blood vessels, which can relieve the pain of arthritis and speed the healing of sprains, strains, and muscle pain. For an athlete, this increase in blood circulation means more oxygen going to muscles. The oxygen promotes glycogen supply to the muscles' energy reserves. Aching and injured muscles recover faster because increased circulation carries off metabolic waste products.

A sauna also acts as a cleansing process for the skin. It improves circulation, which in turn encourages a healthy flow of nutrients to the skin, enhancing tone, texture, and color. You will acquire a new inner glow because your skin is immaculately clean, free of accumulated dirt and dry skin cells. The result: a radiant and younger-looking skin. According to Finnish folklore, "women look their most beautiful an hour after a sauna."

A Few Guidelines

- Consult your physician if you have any health problems to determine if a sauna is safe for you.
- Wait at least two hours after eating before you sauna.
- If you shower before your sauna, you may sweat more; try it with and without first showering to see which you prefer.
- Don't drink alcohol before or immediately after a sauna.
- If this is your first experience with a sauna, stay in for just ten minutes at a time; then follow with a cold shower. Once you make the sauna a regular part of your routine, you may increase your stay as your body becomes more accustomed to its effects.
- Eating a piece of fruit after your sauna session helps replace potassium.
- At the first sign of a cold or flu, increase your sauna sessions. They may be beneficial in boosting your immune system and decreasing the reproductive rate of the viruses.
- Drink plenty of water (at least two eight-

ounce glasses) before and after your stay in the sauna.

CAUTION: In Finland it's not uncommon for doctors to recommend saunas to pregnant women from conception all the way up to the day of delivery. In fact, in Finland saunas were once a traditional place for childbirth. However, in the United States there's a lot of concern about pregnant women taking steam baths or saunas. As a general rule, then, pregnant women and people who have heart disease or have been using drugs or alcohol should stay out of the sauna. Children should not be in saunas without supervision.

EAR CONING

Ear coning has long been used in ancient China, Tibet, and other Eastern countries and has recently been gaining popularity in the West. Ear cones, or ear candles, are used to rid the ears of built-up toxins. Many health practitioners, such as colonic therapists, nutritional consultants, and iridologists, have been recommending the use of ear cones for many years. It is less expensive and easier on the body than other forms of ear cleaning. Reports have noted benefits obtained after the first use of the ear cone as well as further benefits from regular use.

Ear cones are made by taking fine, natural cotton or gauze, spiraling it on a rod, and dipping it in wax. When the large end of the cone is lit and the small end of the cone is positioned in the ear, the smoke filters into the ear canal, warming the ear wax. As the oxygen in the ear is absorbed by the flame, a gentle vacuum is produced, pulling out the excess wax or foreign material from the ear canal and capturing it in the stem of the ear cone. After the procedure and when the flame is extinguished, the cone can be cut with scissors and the wax or debris can be seen. The soft, powdery material in the ear cone will be from the wax and the cloth used to make the cone; the other material is the excess wax that was sucked out of the ear.

There are ear cones on the market which are made of either paraffin or beeswax. Paraffin is a waxy mixture of hydrocarbons distilled from petroleum while beeswax is in its natural form from the hive. Ear candles made of beeswax should obviously be your first choice.

CAUTION: There are ear candles specifically designed for this purpose that can be bought at most health food stores. However, you may wish to consult your physician regarding ear cone candles. This is a two-person procedure. Do not try it alone. Ear cones are not considered a medical device and should not be used if there are surgically placed wires, tubes, or other medical devices in your ear.

WATER

> *Praised be my Lord, for our sister water.*
> *—St. Francis of Assisi,*
> Canticle of the Sun

Replenishing your body with fresh, clean water is essential to the detoxification program. Here's why. Our bodies are mostly water: 20 percent of our bones, 70 percent of our brains, 80 percent of our blood. Yet we use and lose more than two quarts of water every day. For example, the kidneys filter blood plasma (which is predominantly water) all the time. This cleans out the liquid waste and regulates electrolyte levels.

Sodium, potassium, magnesium, and hydrogen are all electrolytes and can be found in lots of different foods, so if your diet is healthy, there is no need for supplements. However, electrolytes need to be continuously replaced by water because they are continually excreted from the body.

In addition, water controls the body's temperature. It carries nutrients and gases around the body. It transports waste products out of the body, lubricates the joints, and keeps the blood "runny." It also helps alleviate toxins through lymphatic drainage. If you want a peaches and cream complexion, drink plenty of water.

How much? At least eight glasses each day. Even slight dehydration will toxify your body, impair your concentration, and give you negative reactions to the world around you.

EXERCISE

During thirty minutes of exercise, you not only burn fat but also lower cholesterol levels, build muscle and bone, detox through the skin and eliminative organs, and improve mental health. It's not necessary to spend your time gyrating in a gym to accomplish all this; what's important is getting active. Exercise is one of the best ways to clean out your system and release those "feel good" endorphins.

"You don't have to work out for days before exercise makes you feel good," says Robert E. Thayer, professor of psychology at California State University, Long Beach. "A simple walk, for example, offers immediate gratification when your mood needs a lift." A study by Thayer's research team found that a brisk ten-minute walk elevated energy and reduced tension (traits associated with being in a good mood) *immediately* and kept doing so for at least sixty minutes following the walk.

Consider this too: Scientists now believe that lifelong physical exertion protects against cancer and diabetes. Researchers at the American Association for the Advancement of Science reported that women who exercised cut their risk of breast and uterine cancer in half and of the most common form of diabetes by two-thirds. Says Harvard reproductive biologist Rose Frisch, who led the 5,398-woman study: "The long-term effects of exercise on health are impressive."

Evidence is also mounting that regular exercise helps protect against colon cancer. Recently a team of researchers at Harvard University's School of Public Health reviewed the exercise habits of seventeen thousand male Harvard alumni who are part of a survey begun in 1962. They found that those who burned one thousand calories or more per week through moderate exercise were half as likely to contract colon cancer as those who didn't. "The theory for *why* exercise reduces the colon cancer risk," says Min Lee, the head of the research team, "is that when people exercise, food passes through the gut faster, minimizing the colon's exposure to any carcinogens."

Another study conducted at Loma Linda University in California showed that even moderate exercise boosts the immune system. After fifteen weeks a group of moderately sedentary women who began a program of exercise showed beneficial changes in their blood cells; there was a 20 percent jump in compounds developed to fight germs. The exercising women also had fewer days of cold symptoms compared with nonexercisers.

Exercise is good at turning negative thoughts into positive energy. Not surprisingly, some of the best evidence comes from Scandinavia, where bleak winters raise the risk of melancholy. In Norway, for example, military recruits are unusually vulnerable to depression during basic training, where they're exiled to the dark and frigid north. K. Gunnar Gotestam, of the University of Tronheim, wondered if exercise could help. He tracked recruits for twelve weeks and found that those who participated in sports during off hours had almost no slump in mood.

In the United States the National Health and Nutrition Examination Survey found that physically active people were half as likely to be depressed a decade later as those who were inactive.

However, as healthy as exercise may be, it's unrealistic to think that you will immediately develop a love affair with it; at its worst exercise is so boring it can drive you to fantasize about spending the rest of your life on the couch, eating bonbons, and channel surfing. That's why it's imperative to choose an exercise program that fits well with your temperament (if you're not a social person, for example, don't choose an aerobics class; opt for walking instead) and to try to vary your exercise program as much as possible to avoid burnout.

Popular Options and Their Benefits

BIKING

For an aerobic sport that promises little stress on joints but plenty of scenery, try cycling. For a real workout, consider mountain biking. As you crank up the rougher terrain, you'll work your heart harder.

CROSS-COUNTRY SKIING

This winter sport comes in far ahead of downhill skiing (in which momentum does much of the work) and is one of the few aerobic activities that engage most muscles and give you the endorphin rush of being outdoors. Cross-country trails abound in state and national parks, or if you're lucky enough to live in the country, you can make your own trails nearer to home.

DANCING

Whether you take a class or just bop to your favorite rock and roll, you'll earn a terrific cardiovascular workout, and the music keeps you motivated. Don't overlook ballroom, tap, jazz, ballet, or even belly dancing. Just keep moving between songs, and add a lot of arm action to increase your heart rate.

SWIMMING

A terrific nonimpact sport that uses muscles from head to toe, this activity is perfect if your weight makes other types of exercise uncomfortable. To achieve real cardiovascular benefits, you need fast strokes, with little gliding in between. If you can't swim, try aqua aerobics: walking, running in place, even doing jumping jacks while immersed. The water gives your heart and muscles extra resistance to work against yet cushions your joints.

WALKING

Exercise doesn't get any easier than this. Perfect for newcomers to exercise, walking offers all the aerobic advantages of running, but it won't jar your joints. If you want to pump up the fitness factor, just quicken the pace, pump your arms forward and back, and head for the hills or sloping pathways.

How to Find Your Heart Rate

Many exercise experts believe that to ensure fitness, you must perform an activity intensely enough to raise your heart rate to at least 40 percent and perferably between 50 and 85 percent of your maximum heart rate (MHR), your heartbeats per minute. To find your MHR, subtract your age from 220. Then, to find the range of your training heart rate (THR), multiply that number by 0.5 and then 0.85. (For instance, a forty-year-old's MHR is 180; her THR should be between 90 and 153 beats per minute.) You can easily check whether you are reaching your range. During an exercise session, take your pulse for six seconds; multiply the number of beats by ten. Find the level in your range that feels right for you. In time you'll know how it "feels" to work out at your training heart rate, and taking your pulse during each exercise session may not be necessary.

TAI CHI

Tai chi is an ancient Chinese exercise and relaxation technique that helps relieve stress while keeping the joints flexible and the muscles toned. Following on the heels of a study that showed tai chi could reduce falls in the elderly comes a report indicating that the practice also improves cardiovascular fitness after a heart attack. British researchers reporting in the *Postgraduate Medical Journal,* compared how 126 heart attack patients fared in three different cardiac rehabilitation programs: tai chi, aerobic exercise, and a nonexercise support group. At the end of the eight-week trial, only those doing tai chi showed a reduction in resting heart rate and diastolic blood pressure. The researchers concluded that the gentle movements used in tai chi offered the ultimate in relaxation.

Basic Tai Chi Movements

POLISHING THE MIRROR

Standing with your feet apart, imagine you are holding two rags in front of a large mirror. Concentrating on your body movements, place hands side by side above your head and slowly lower them, circling the left hand to the left and the right hand to the right, until your fingertips are at shoulder level. Now proceed to the crouch movement.

CROUCH

With your arms extended at shoulder level, bend your knees, and lower your rear to a squatting position, keeping your back straight. Slowly bring your palms in front of your chest, and stand, maintaining the hand position. Resume polishing the mirror movement. Repeat the entire series five times.

SWING

Stand with your feet together and your upper body relaxed. Flex your left knee, slowly swing your right leg forward until your thigh is parallel to the ground, then slowly swing it back again; continue swinging your leg forward and backward five times. Switch legs and repeat.

AWAKENING THE SENSES

OPEN HEARING

This means listening to the whole range and variety of sound vibrations that surround us. It's not just music that can affect our mood; every noise that enters our soul leaves its mark. If you train yourself to appreciate *all* sounds, you will be less likely to regard noise as an irritation and be more likely to embrace it as a living experience.

Try this exercise: Sit comfortably near a window. Close your eyes, and remain very still until you can hear the noise in your head. Now open up your listening to include sounds in the room.

Follow this by including the sounds in the street outdoors and finally more distant sounds.

OPEN SEEING

Although we all possess a wide field of vision, most of us focus on one small area at a time. Begin to pay attention to your outer or peripheral vision, which will lead you to a wider perspective. Also, pay attention to the behavior of other people and their body language, which may send you subtle messages beyond their verbal cues.

OPEN TASTING

Prepare a meal for yourself, but keep the ingredients separate. Begin to eat the food slowly, savoring the flavor of each mouthful. Pay attention to how your teeth and tongue feel against the textures of the food. Swallow slowly.

OPEN SMELLING

Gather together some strong-smelling objects, like flowers, herbs, fruit, or soap. Close your eyes, and pick up the objects one at a time; allow yourself the opportunity to absorb the fragrance of each item.

OPEN TOUCHING

Select some objects as different in weight and texture as you can find. The collection might include a shell, silk scarf, pumice stone, and piece of ice. The selection is entirely your personal choice, but keep it varied. Place what you have chosen on a tabletop. After closing your eyes, pick up each item in turn, and explore it thoroughly, noticing any differences in textures and temperature. Our sense of touch provides a vital source of information about our "state of being" and is a major source of pleasure. Even everyday tasks like washing your hair can be enriched by attuning to the "feel" of the whole experience rather than doing it mechanically.

MEDITATION

> *What lies behind us and what lies*
> *before us are tiny matters,*
> *compared to what lies within us.*
> —*Ralph Waldo Emerson*

Every moment of our waking lives our minds are running on fast speed, buzzing with innumerable perceptions and worries, working on overdrive. Most of the time we're not aware of our constant humming thoughts even though they can create negative energy and pollute our physical and emotional lives. But as long as our minds are restless, it's impossible to come into true harmony within ourselves.

Once you make meditation a daily habit, communication with the world will become smooth, gentle, and free from friction. Through meditation you can open yourself to the experience of profound well-being because when you reach the center of peace and quiet within yourself, you simply enjoy *being*. You are able to maintain an inner balance, purifying your mind and body.

There's a substantial collection of studies to confirm the benefits of meditation. I've selected only a few:

PAIN MANAGEMENT

Meditation has proved to be an excellent strategy for people coping with headache, backache, and other forms of chronic pain. In one study, researchers found that 72 percent of patients continued to report "moderate to great improvement" three years after learning to meditate.

ANXIETY

Too much stress can trigger panic attacks, depression, and chronic anxiety. In a study at the University of Massachusetts, twenty out of twenty-two anxiety-prone volunteers showed a significant improvement in anxiety scores following an eight-week course in meditation, dropping from an average of twenty (out of twenty-five) to eight.

HIGH BLOOD PRESSURE

In one of the largest and most reliable studies, blood pressure dropped an average of 8 to 10 percent after three months of daily meditation.

IMMUNE SYSTEM

Meditation boosts the immune system and reduces illnesses. When Dr. David Orme-Johnson compared insurance data from two thousand meditators and an equal number of nonmeditators, he found that the meditating group had 90 percent less heart disease, 55 percent fewer tumors, and 30 percent fewer infectious diseases.

PMS

Meditation can help alleviate such premenstrual symptoms as fatigue, depression, water retention, and insomnia. In one study, women with severe PMS showed a 58 percent improvement after five months of daily meditation.

Although meditation has profound effects on our well-being, it doesn't have to be a complicated process. Advanced meditators may prefer to sit on a cushion in a lotus or half-lotus position and focus on their breathing or on a particular chakra (as discussed in Chapter 2). But for beginners, follow these basic steps:

1. Sit in a quiet, comfortable place on a straight-back chair or floor cushion. Relax your muscles, but do not lie down.
2. Select a syllable, phrase, or word, such as "one," "peace," "love," or "om" to focus on.
3. Close your eyes and follow the rhythm of your breathing, relaxing a little bit more with each breath.
4. Repeat your chosen word as you breathe in and out. If your mind wanders, don't quit. Just let your thoughts go, and refocus by repeating your chosen word.
5. Continue for ten to twenty minutes (pick the length of time beforehand, and stick to it). You may open your eyes occasionally to check the time, but don't use an alarm; it's too jarring.

When you finish, sit quietly for a minute or two—first with eyes closed, then with eyes open. Allow yourself to imagine turning your home and office into a peaceful, toxic-free retreat and your bathroom into an all-natural home spa.

Read on.

6

Complete Your Detox: Create a Safe Haven and a Natural Home Spa

*It is not because things are
difficult that we do not dare;
it is because we do not dare that
they are difficult.*
—Seneca

Most of us spend at least 90 percent of our lives indoors, but too often our homes and workplaces are toxic environments that compromise our immune systems and leave us feeling deenergized and depressed. The catch-22 is that after a detox fast, the body is more sensitive than ever to pollutants; it becomes a "virgin" host to toxins. But it's not a hopeless situation. In this chapter you'll learn about the important steps you can take to eliminate toxic elements in your home and your work space.

It may seem like a lot of time and effort to reorganize your environment, but consider it "wellspring" cleaning. Once it is accomplished, you will immediately feel energy surge through your environment. The desire to spend more peaceful, introspective time in your home will increase; clear thinking and more focused production at your workplace will also be apparent.

AT HOME

In the Kitchen: Check Out Your Cleaners

Many chemicals contained in common cleaners are toxic, but this doesn't mean you have to forgo a spick-and-span kitchen. Most health food stores stock nontoxic alternatives, or you can buy them through mail-order companies, like the Seventh Generation catalog (1-800-456-1177). Here are a few do-it-yourself cleaners:

• To clear away grease and eliminate odors, I use the all-purpose cleaner baking soda. It works as a gentle scouring powder. Just sprinkle it on a damp sponge, and clean your countertops, sinks, bathrooms, tubs, and even ovens. Use baking soda to eliminate odors from dish towels and other cleaning cloths by adding a cupful to your laundry instead of bleach.

• Don't use supermarket dish soaps; they're loaded with petroleum-based cleansers, artificial dyes, and synthetic fragrances. Instead use the cleaning power of natural cleansers like olive oil, as well as the fragrance and grease-cutting power of essential oils (such as lemon and tea tree) and natural skin smoothers like aloe.

• To shine your furniture, use a natural furniture polish by mixing one teaspoon of olive oil with one-fourth cup of vinegar. I usually mix up a batch and store it in a tightly sealed jar.

• For a natural disinfectant, mix two tablespoons of tea tree oil with two cups of water, and pour it into a spray bottle.

• Use only cellulose sponges for keeping countertops clean. Toss them into your dishwasher once a week to keep them germ-free. Be sure to change sponges at least every two months so bacteria don't build up.

• To scrub dishes, pots, and pans, use untreated copper scouring pads or natural bristle brushes. Replace these every two months as well.

• Use iron or ceramic rather than harmful

aluminum pots that may leave toxic aluminum residues on your foods.

• Change from a gas oven and stove to an electric one. According to a recent British study, women who cook with gas stoves have an increased risk of asthma. Researchers advise asthmatic women who cook with gas to make sure their kitchens are adequately ventilated and, if possible, to get an electric stove.

• Have your water tested. If toxins are found, or the water is chlorinated, filter the drinking water or use bottled water.

Make Your Living Room Breathable

• It pays to wipe your feet before coming into the house. Even better, leave your shoes at the door, and keep a pair of natural fabric slippers on a mat. A recent study sponsored by the Environmental Protection Agency (EPA) found that a commonly used lawn weed killer is readily carried on the soles of people's shoes into homes, where it settles into carpets and poses a possible hazard to small children and susceptible adults. Taking your shoes off at the door cuts track-in pollutants by about 90 percent.

• When a house remains at a steady, cool temperature, there is less likelihood of molds and mildew developing. To accomplish this, increase southern and eastern light into your home during the summer months. It's not as hot as afternoon light and therefore keeps your home cooler.

• Try to dust at least once a week. As many as two thousand dust mites can live in a single teaspoon of dust. Allergy product stores sell dust mite–resistant chair and couch covers (call the Asthma and Allergy Foundation of America at 1-800-7-ASTHMA for a list of mail-order companies).

• Ventilate. Lack of ventilation not only can make you feel lethargic but can also lead to more serious respiratory problems. Give your ventilation system a once-over every month or so. Check air filters, drain pans, and cooling coils to ensure they are working properly. Ventilation grilles should not be blocked by furniture.

• Clean your carpets. Wall-to-wall carpets are notorious allergen trappers. Shampoo (with nontoxic detergent) regularly, and keep the carpets well aired. If you're buying a new rug, choose a washable one made from natural fibers (synthetic materials give off noxious fumes), and ask to see the manufacturer's notes on emissions.

• Consider using linoleum made from all-natural materials (not synthetic linoleum, which contains chemicals) instead of carpeting.

• Keep your home at a relative humidity of 30 to 50 percent.

• If the inside of your home contains lead-based paint, have it removed by a certified professional. The fee will run from one hundred to one thousand dollars or more, depending on the size of your house and how much lead needs to be removed. To find a professional, call the local U.S. Department of Housing and Development office.

• If you have miniblinds, check the label to see if they were made in Taiwan, China, or Mexico. If so, run a home test kit (available at home improvement stores) on the blinds. If lead is found, remove the blinds.

• Test to see if your house's exterior paint is lead-based. You can keep lead dust from being tracked inside by placing a mat at entrances and asking guests to wipe their shoes or, better yet, to remove them.

• The U.S. Health and Human Services Department recommends that everyone measure the levels of radon in his or her house. Passive monitors are available for radon, formaldehyde, nitrogen dioxide, and water vapor. You can install one of these devices and leave it in your home to detect certain pollutants. Over time you will need to send the device to a laboratory to be analyzed. Monitors for each pollutant with laboratory analysis cost between fifteen and fifty dollars. Organizations such as the American Society of Heating, Refrigerating and Air-Conditioning Engineers, the World Health Organization, and the American Council of Government and Industrial Hygienists can offer guidance to what levels of indoor pollution may be harmful to your health.

• If you decide to have your home tested for indoor pollution, your state or local health office may be able to refer you to air-quality experts equipped to perform the testing. These experts can test your home for various pollutants, measure infiltration rates, and advise you on the need to control further and reduce levels of pollution. Your regional EPA office can supply additional information on indoor pollution.

Create a Dream Bedroom

• Always choose cotton or silk sheets rather than polyester or synthetic blends. Most polyester sheets on the market today are coated with a formaldehyde finish, which allows the sheets to resist wrinkling. Formaldehyde fumes are released for the life of your sheets; they don't wash out in the laundry.

• Use cotton-filled pillows rather than chemically drenched polyester foam. For non-toxic pillows that offer substantial back and neck support, try buckwheat hull pillows. They conform to the shape of your neck and head to relieve and avoid muscle strain while you sleep.

• Most curtains today, like carpets, are made from chemical-emitting polyesters. Untreated cotton curtains are the best coverage for your windows. These range from light-weight to long, sunlight-blocking drapes. It's also better to buy vegetable-dyed cotton than chemically colored fabrics.

• In the warm summer months most experts agree that you should sleep without clothes. When you don't wear clothes to bed, you give your skin a chance to breathe. In cooler months, when you need a little extra insulation, choose sleepwear made from natural fabrics.

• Electromagnetic fields, the invisible forces produced by electricity and emitted by electrical appliances, have been linked to serious health problems, from brain tumors to breast cancer. To protect yourself, keep TVs, computers, electric heaters, electric clocks, and other electrical appliances at least three feet from your bed. Beyond that distance EMFs drop off rapidly. Electric alarm clocks, particularly the old, dial-faced models, are notorious EMF emitters; use battery or sun-operated alarms. Electric blankets are even more dangerous because they remain plugged in (and hot) and lie directly over your body for hours on end. Untreated, natural down-filled blankets are an excellent substitute.

• Stick to furnishing your bedroom with your grandmother's old chests, wicker, rod iron, or hardwood pieces. Today most affordable bedroom furniture—including bed frames—is constructed from a material known as particleboard, which is pressed wood shavings held together with unreaformaldehyde resin.

• The air you breathe all night should be as pure as possible. Common houseplants make attractive and soothing natural air purifiers. To keep the air fresh, sleep with your window opened just a crack, even in the winter. This way air circulates, gases dissipate, and the humidity is maintained.

• Finally, make your bedroom a perfect place to relax, dream, and make love. If there's something in your room that jars your sensibility, take it out. Keep by your bedside your journal, candles, incense, a lavender sachet under your pillow (to induce sleep and enhance dreaming), an absorbing novel, and massage oils. My astrologer, Pam Ciampi, also suggests placing a small bowl of salt water on your night table to soak up negative vibrations.

Use Nontoxic Pest Control

• Never use potent insect repellants. Certain clothing colors are less likely to invite insects to you than others. Stick with white, tan, khaki, and light green. Also, mosquitoes are often attracted to certain commercial deodorants, hair sprays, and shaving lotions. When you go outdoors, go natural. Tie some thyme, basil, lavender, or mint on your hat to repel flying insects.

• If your house gets infested with ants, put dried coffee grounds around the doors leading to the kitchen, and sprinkle red pepper in your cabinet and on your countertops.

• Don't use mothballs. In addition to being highly toxic, mothballs can't kill moth eggs already in clothing. Wash your wardrobe carefully before storing it for the winter.

• Much safer and perhaps more effective than commercial pesticides in stopping wasps, bees, and roaches is hair spray, which immobilizes insects, especially winged ones. Use a pump bottle; never use an aerosol can that contains toxic chemicals that contribute to the destruction of the earth's ozone layer.

• If mealworms get into your open packages of noodles, rice, or flour, place a wrapped stick of spearmint chewing gum next to the packages.

Nontoxic Pet Care

• Never flea bomb your house. The safest bet if your animal has fleas is to use a commercial shampoo; it has not been shown to cause any nerve poison or skin irritation. Opt for a fatty acid soap that can be bought at a pet shop or a garden supply store. You can also fight the flea wars by dabbing petroleum jelly on a flea comb and running it through your pet's fur. The fleas should stick to the comb. Make sure to drown them in warm water, and then clean the comb carefully with soapy water.

• Look for flea sprays that contain methoprene and hydropene, as opposed to those that contain limonene. Or simply try sprinkling talcum powder on your pet to kill fleas. The best time to treat your pets is *before* flea season in the spring. Be diligent.

• If your home becomes infested with fleas, sprinkle your carpet with salt and then vacuum a day later. The salt will dehydrate the fleas.

This method is simple and very effective. Be sure to remove the bag from your vacuum cleaner when you're through; then seal and dispose of it.

• You can also try mixing brewer's yeast or primrose oil with your pet's dinner. These additives will help keep your animal's skin healthy, moist, and unattractive to fleas since fleas are attracted to chapped and dry coats. Pet owners I know have sworn by these additives, although my dog just walks away from his bowl when I've tried them. Good luck.

• Use only a ceramic feeding bowl. Bacteria can hide in the porous surfaces of plastic.

IN YOUR OFFICE

A nagging cold that magically disappears when you leave your office may actually be sick building syndrome, and according to the American Lung Association, thousands of Americans are affected each year. The symptoms include headaches, dizziness, breathing difficulties, and eye, nose, and throat irritation.

Obviously, if you're not working in a home office, your ability to change the physical conditions of your environment may be limited. But if you believe your office is toxic, you may diplomatically want to identify the culprits to management and offer some methods to remedy the situation.

To begin with, building materials are responsible for a considerable amount of indoor air pollution. Some paints, adhesives, pressed-wood products, and glues (fused in carpets) release volatile organic compounds (VOCs), pollutants that become gases at room temperature.

If your company has just had a new carpet installed, ask management to open windows to increase ventilation. Ideally, it should install the carpeting on a weekend. Also, ask the management to place copy machines near an open window so that ozone emissions drift right outside.

The ventilation system should be checked regularly. Ventilation systems in large buildings are designed not only to heat and cool the air but also to draw in and circulate outdoor air. Unfortunately, companies often turn down the systems to save money. In older or poorly maintained buildings, blocked vents can trap stale air. Poor ventilation can lead to headaches, nausea, fatigue, dry skin, concentration problems, and eye, nose, and throat irritations.

The American Society of Heating, Refrigerating and Air-Conditioning Engineers recommends a circulation of fifteen to sixty cubic feet of outside air per minute for each employee. If air circulation is blocked by partitions, you should suggest they be raised at least six inches off the floor.

To give credibility to your concerns, ask for the free pamphlet *Indoor Air Pollution in the Office* from the American Lung Association at 1-800-LUNG-USA, and contact the Indoor Air Quality Information Clearinghouse at 1-800-438-4318 for free copies of the EPA fact sheets "Sick Building Syndrome" and "Ventilation and Air Quality in Offices."

You might consider buying a portable air filter for your car and plugging it in at your desk with a converter unit. And speak to your boss about installing a tinted radiation screen for your computer terminal; it eases eyestrain, increases productivity, and screens out harmful EMFs.

Also, bring your own coffee mug; you'll reduce waste and won't be drinking out of plastic. Ask the office manager whether it's possible to buy organic coffee and unbleached coffee filters or a coffeemaker that doesn't use disposable filters. Ideally, you have already cut back on your coffee intake thanks to your detox fast.

If you're lucky enough to have a home office, you can create a personal space that is not only nontoxic but also emotionally and creatively enriching; the possibilities are all your own. For example, I keep a meditation pillow in my office for those times when my mind is so busy that I can't settle down and concentrate. I also find that burning incense before I begin work at my desk helps me focus and center. Also within reach are books of spiritual encouragement, like Anne Lamott's *Bird by Bird* and Julia Cameron's *The Artist's Way*. I break frequently to give myself a shoulder massage, stretch, play a game of ring toss, or read a poem. Rather than think of work as a chore, I try (even when the pressure is on) to consider it a blessing, and I give thanks for the joy of accomplishment.

And at the end of my day I know what is usually awaiting: an hour's worth of heaven on earth—my own natural home spa.

TURN YOUR BATHROOM INTO A NATURAL HOME SPA

After a hard day of work, unwind and rejuvenate yourself in your own tranquil refuge. It's easy to do, and the payoff is immeasurable. Between 7:00 and 8:00 P.M., at least three times a week, I retreat to my personal "sanctum sanitarium." My family knows that unless it's an emergency, I am to be left alone, *undisturbed.* Truthfully, this practice took some training, but now they've come to appreciate the relaxed and open woman who emerges after her spa session;

they gladly leave me in peace. Let the rich and famous pay extravagant sums to be wrapped, buffed, and smoothed at a luxury spa, I have it all in my own time and in my own home. And so can you. Don't feel that it's impossible to set this kind of time aside for yourself. *Consider your spa sessions a mandatory element in your detoxing program.*

To create a spa atmosphere, stock up on the following soothing essentials:

—Plenty of candles, preferably votive or natural beeswax
—Massage oils*
—Facial masks
—Bath soothers
—Slougher
—Pumice stone
—Natural botanic shampoo
—Tape of your favorite relaxing music
—Bottles of spring water
—Thick undyed cotton towels
—Cozy cotton bathrobe

* Recipes follow.

Set the Stage

Turn on your tape machine with the volume at low. Light several small votive candles (scented if you prefer), and place them strategically so that their reflection flickers on the water. Slowly undress while watching yourself in the mirror. Think positive thoughts about your body. If you find yourself dwelling on a body part you don't like, tell yourself, "That's not the whole picture of my being." And affirm: "Although my body is the temple of my soul, it is the true nature of my soul that projects outward."

Since your time is precious, you want to opt for the treatment that suits your particular need for the day. When you have the right attitude, just bathing is a grand sensual experience, and you can simply drizzle one or two teaspoons of your favorite fragrant oil (lavender, patchouli, musk, rose, almond, or vanilla) for an overall aromatic experience, or you can choose one of these specific bathing remedies:

DETOXING AROMATHERAPY BATH

Cut the leg from a clean pair of panty hose; fill with with one tablespoon each of dried chamomile and rosemary and four drops of lavender oil. Knot open one end to form a sachet; then tie it under the faucet so that the water runs through.

182

Fill the tub with warm water; soak for thirty minutes, sipping from your bottle of spring water. The herbs have a calming effect, while the water temperature raises body heat and eliminates impurities.

MUSCLE RELAXING BATH

Mix together one-third cup of baking soda, one-fourth cup of citric acid crystals or powder (available in most supermarkets or the vitamin section of your pharmacy), and one tablespoon of cornstarch. Place in a tight-fitting dry glass jar. (This should yield about ten tubfuls.) Fill your bath with warm water, and sprinkle two tablespoons into the water. Enjoy the invigorating fizz and bubble for twenty minutes. While you soak, try some progressive relaxation. Begin by letting your feet float on the surface of the bathwater. To do this, your feet must be completely relaxed. Feel that relaxation slowly migrate up your body to your head.

SLIMMING BATH (EASES WATER RETENTION)

Mix together juniper/lemon or sandalwood/ geranium in olive oil. Put twenty drops of each in a tub of warm water. These essential oils not only smooth and tone your skin but can help release the water buildup in your tissues.

QUICK TIP: If your feet are swollen, soak them in

a basin of lukewarm water containing six drops of juniper and four drops of lemon oil. Use a pumice stone to remove dry skin and soften calluses. Then massage your feet and ankles with upward strokes.

SUPER STRESS-BUSTING BATH

Brew one cup of chamomile tea, and let cool. Add five drops of marjoram oil and ten drops of lavender oil. Add to the bath. While you're soaking, practice some deep breathing: Inhale and exhale slowly, focusing on each breath.

ROMANTIC SOAK

When you're in the mood for love, combine one-half cup of rosebuds and five whole dried cloves, placed in a sachet as described in the "Detoxing Aromatherapy Bath." Rose is the ultimate fragrance of romance and has certain aphrodisiac qualities, stimulating feelings of sensuality and sexual responsiveness. Cloves will add a dash of spice and zestiness to your lovemaking.

Regardless of the bath treatment you choose, before adding these mixtures to the bath, apply to a small area of skin to test for sensitivity. Always enter the tub slowly, even gracefully, trying hard not to disturb the water. You might want to prop your head up with a pillow or just lie back; let the world float into oblivion.

When you're ready to get out of the tub, wait a few more minutes for some serious sloughing. You want to remove dead skin cells and leave your skin porous and fresh. There are lots of ways to slough. But I recommend using either a natural sea sponge, which has a soothing, slightly abrasive texture, a natural wool fiber mitt, or a soft, natural-fiber bath brush, all of which exfoliate gently.

When you're through, leave the tub as gracefully as you entered. Wrap yourself in a big towel. You're relaxed and at peace and it's now time to choose another natural spa option.

Après-Tub Treatments

SOOTHING HAND SOAK

To smooth and soothe dry, rough skin and nails, soak your hands in a little warm vegetable or castor oil, and follow with this healing massage: Mix two parts of boiled oatmeal with equal amounts of rose water and milk (enough to make a paste), and add two drops of glycerin. Rub the mixture on your hands for several minutes; then rinse. Give yourself some applause; you now have the hands of a twenty-year-old.

BODY SCRUBBER

To help make your skin silky, mix one-fourth cup of salt with one-half cup of olive oil. Rub the mixture over your clean, dry skin in a circular motion, using a soft body sponge (not a scruffy loofah). Rinse with tepid water, and gently pat your skin dry.

LYMPHATIC DRAINAGE SELF-MASSAGE

When your body is warm and your skin is receptive, it's a great time for concentrating on lymphatic drainage. Pour about one teaspoon of sesame oil and a drop of your favorite scent into your hands, and sweep them over your chest and buttocks. Use firm upward strokes. Not only does upward sweeping tone the breast tissues, but it drains toxins into the lymph nodes under the armpits. The breast is made up of glandular tissues, and draining them can prevent mastitis and other diseases caused by breast congestion.

Continue your massage by oiling your legs, arms, neck, shoulders, and torso. Sweep upward to drain the arms and legs, using your fingers to massage your thighs, neck, and shoulders. Pay special attention to your solar plexus, the area between your breast and stomach that is a storage center of nervous energy. Circle the solar plexus at least six times, inhaling the fragrance of the oils as you work.

If you use a light base, such as sesame, your oil should be quickly absorbed and you should be able to wrap yourself in a cozy bathrobe. However, if you feel a little oily, give yourself a quick rubdown with a natural cotton towel.

HYDRATING BODY WRAP

Heat is the secret ingredient in this intensive moisturizing treatment. After your bath and exfoliation, pat your skin dry, and slather on a moisturizer, preferably a natural oil, from the neck down. Place four towels in the dryer; heat them for three to five minutes, and set two of them on the bed. Lie on two of the towels, and cover yourself with the other two. Relax for thirty minutes. I like to listen to my favorite CD, read a good novel, or visualize lying on a tropical beach. When finished, rise slowly, and towel off any excess moisturizer. Spritz on some soothing lavender mist (fill a misting bottle with distilled water and a few drops of lavender oil).

BODY MASK

This thick amber-toned mask contains fragrant sage and thyme leaves, which are natural stimulants, plus almond and peppermint essences to stimulate your senses and moisturize your skin; black tea and honey work to tone, refresh, and condition your skin (black tea is a soother and astringent; honey is a humectant).

2½	cups water
4	black tea bags
2	tablespoons chopped fresh sage leaves
2	tablespoons fresh thyme leaves
1	teaspoon pectin
1	teaspoon honey
½	teaspoon almond extract
½	teaspoon peppermint extract

Bring the water to a boil. Immerse the tea bags, sage, and thyme in the water, reduce the heat, and let simmer for twenty minutes. Remove from heat, and allow to cool slightly. Remove tea bags, and stir in pectin, honey, and extracts. Refrigerate mixture for eight to twelve hours, or until it achieves a gelatinous consistency.

Apply the mask to your body. Leave it on for fifteen minutes; then rinse in a warm shower. The mask will keep for five days if it is covered and refrigerated.*

* Adapted from Philip B., *Blended Beauty: Botanical Secrets for Body & Soul*. Used by permission of Ten Speed Press, Berkeley, California.

INVIGORATING SELF-MASSAGE (for nights on the town)

A massage not only relaxes, but can help your body come alive all over. Enjoy moisturizing and aromatherapeutic benefits by pouring one-half cup of jojoba, canola, or sweet almond oil into a clean pitcher or container and then adding the following:

- 15 drops rosemary oil
- 10 drops lavender oil
- 5 drops geranium oil
- 5 drops grapefruit oil
- 3 drops basil oil
- 2 drops peppermint oil

Stir or shake gently to blend. Massage onto arms, legs, feet, and shoulders with your finger-tips, using circular motions and light pressure.

Facial Treatments

Many of the facial treatments described below can be applied while you're still soaking in the tub. In fact, a mask will work even better if you apply it while bathing because the steam rising from the tub works to open your pores.

EXFOLIATING PASTE

To rejuvenate skin, mix two teaspoons of oatmeal, two teaspoons of ground almonds, and two teaspoons of grated lemon peel. Add water to make a paste; then massage the paste into your skin gently to remove dead cells and expose healthy new skin below. Rinse with warm water.

CUCUMBER FACIAL SCRUB

In a blender puree one-half cup of peeled and chopped cucumbers. Add one tablespoon of baking soda, one egg, and two tablespoons of plain yogurt; blend on medium-low setting for two minutes. Apply in gentle circular motions to your moistened face. When finished, rinse your face with warm water. (You might choose to prepare this scrub in advance; if refrigerated, it will stay fresh up to four days.)

STRAWBERRY PORE MINIMIZER

Strawberries act as an astringent to minimize pores and help slough off dry skin. This unique treatment was originally developed at the Sanibel Harbor Resort & Spa in Fort Myers, Florida: Place a layer of gauze on your face, and cover it with six to eight sliced fresh (preferably organic) strawberries. Leave on for twenty minutes, and then rinse with cool spring water.

NUTRITIOUS SKIN SOFTENER

Mash one-half banana with two tablespoons of sunflower oil. Pop open a vitamin E capsule, and add the contents to your paste. Smooth the paste over your clean, dry face, and leave on as you would a mask for twenty minutes. Rinse gently with warm water, and pat dry.

SIMPLE ANTIOXIDANT MASK

Steam one large carrot, and mash it thoroughly. To achieve a pasty consistency, add a small amount of water. Apply to the face for ten minutes; then rinse off.

YOGURT COOLING MASK

Mix three teaspoons of plain organic yogurt (a natural cleanser and nourisher) and three tablespoons of honey (which locks in moisture). Smooth onto your clean skin, and leave on for fifteen minutes. Remove with cool spring water. Now apply pure aloe vera juice with a cotton ball. Aloe vera not only cleanses your skin but also heals and detoxifies it.

SEAWEED SKIN SAVER

Rehydrate a few strips of dry seaweed by soaking them in tepid water for twenty minutes. Rub the seaweed over your face, using either a washcloth or your fingers for a few minutes; then splash your face with cool water. For a more intensive once-a-week treatment, apply several strips of rinsed fresh or rehydrated seaweed to your face; relax for twenty to thirty minutes; then rinse off.

WRINKLE REMEDIES

Red wine is an ancient Roman remedy for wrinkled, older skin; the wine contains a natural acid that smooths superficial lines. Mix one tablespoon of red wine with two tablespoons of honey. Smooth it onto your face, and allow it to dry; then rinse. Be sure to follow up with a moisturizer with antiaging emollients like jojoba, cocoa butter, olive oil, or aloe vera.

Or mix one-half cup of mashed pineapple with one tablespoon of honey, and apply the mixture to your face. Relax for ten minutes, and then wash with cool water.

Brewer's yeast is also touted as effective in smoothing skin and minimizing laugh lines. Make a paste with brewer's yeast and avocado oil. Allow it to dry completely before rinsing off your face.

MIGHTY MOISTURIZER

In India women keep their complexions glowing with rose water, sprayed lightly on the face and allowed to dry, followed with a bit of clarified butter, which moisturizes and protects the skin.

This works especially well for dry complexions but may be too rich a moisturizer for oily complexions.

Hair Treatments

SUPERCONDITIONING HAIR PACK

It's best if you can apply this or a similar treatment to your hair at least once a week. This conditioning hair pack is one of my favorites because all the ingredients come from my kitchen: Mix together one-half cup of mayonnaise, one-half of a mashed ripe avocado, and two teaspoons of lemon juice. Rinse your hair with warm water; then apply the hair pack. Cover your hair with a plastic bag or old shower cap, and leave on for fifteen minutes. Shampoo out.

AROMATIC HAIR SHINER

In a small pot, heat one-quarter cup of almond oil until it's comfortably warm. Mix in five drops each of chamomile, lavender, and patchouli essential oils. Once the mixture has cooled to a comfortable temperature, apply it to your clean, damp hair. After fifteen minutes, shampoo until you get a good, vigorous lather going, then rinse.

SPA SHAMPOO FOR OILY HAIR

Mix your own shampoo by adding ten drops of juniper, cypress, or lemon oil with a cup of mild, unscented soap. All these oils are effective astringents that should help stimulate as well as dry an oily scalp.

REVERSAL HAIR RINSE

Add three drops of jojoba oil to your favorite botanic shampoo. Then choose the rinse that suits your hair's needs: Cider vinegar is good for proper pH balance, egg yolk for body, and coconut oil for shine. After applying the rinse, shampoo again; then repeat the rinse.

DRY AND BRITTLE HAIR REMEDY

Apply mayonnaise to either wet or dry hair for thirty minutes; then shampoo it out. Repeat the procedure no more than once a week.

DANDRUFF DESTROYER

Dandruff is characterized by an excessive sloughing of the scalp's skin cells and is often caused by stress, dietary imbalances, and overuse of commercial shampoos. The most effective and easiest remedy is to massage your scalp with vegetable oil before shampooing. The oil will help soften and loosen dandruff flakes. Wash out with a botanical shampoo, and follow with a rinse of apple cider vinegar diluted in warm water.

Natural Grooming Potpourri

SENSIBLE CELLULITE TREATMENT

Cellulite is plain old fat that has bunched up in little pockets. The popular procedure of vacuuming appeals more to vanity than good health. Whether or not this mechanical shortcut holds lasting results is still open to debate. But if you are really serious about shedding cellulite, eat plenty of fresh fruits and vegetables, which detoxify the body, and drink lots of water. Top nutritionists say people with cellulite don't drink enough water. Six to eight glasses of water per day (minimum) tend to open up the blood vessels just below the skin level where most cellulite hides and helps flush it out. At the same time, reduce the salt in your diet. Salt makes your body retain water and adds to the cellulite condition. Some light muscle-building workouts tone up the tissues where cellulite ordinarily collects, so it doesn't have room to form. Meanwhile, reinforce exercise by dry brushing your skin with rosemary, sandalwood, juniper, or lemon oil dabbed on a brush. Any one of these essences will penetrate the skin and work to improve circulation and detoxify. Although it's good to massage cellulite-prone areas like the buttocks and thighs, go easy on the skin. Cellulite-dappled spots are usually very tender. Brush gently until pink, take a bath with one of the detox formulas, and then massage the cellulite area again.

INSTANT SHIATSU FACE-LIFT

Put your fingers near the center of your cheeks, at the place where the bone protrudes, and move them down slightly, then slightly out toward your ears. Stimulating these points can increase circulation and relax the drawn or fatigued areas around the mouth and eyes, soothing fatigued eyes and reducing puffiness.

STRETCH MARK STOPPER

It's true. Vitamin E oil or cream applied to stretch marks and scars will help soften and relieve them.

PUFFY EYE SOOTHER

I tend to get puffy eyes, probably because of too little sleep. As a remedy, once a week I incorporate this treatment into my spa time: Grate a few teaspoons of fresh cucumber on two cotton pads, or steep, then cool two chamomile tea bags, and place them on your eyes for twenty minutes.

GLOSSIER EYELASHES

Use a bit of petroleum jelly on your eyelash curler, or curl your lashes on the back of a spoon.

THROAT MOISTURIZER

This is where age really shows, and we often neglect moisturizing the neck. For especially dry or dehydrated skin, apply some warm peanut oil, and massage upward along the neck.

HAIR SETTER

Flat beer and milk are great hair setters; if your hair is oily, use skim milk.

PIMPLE AND BLACKHEAD CURES

Fight back as soon as a pimple becomes visible but not with toxic cortisone creams. Instead apply ice for five or six seconds every half hour; this will often stop the pimple within a couple of hours. Or dab individual pimples with a bit of tea tree oil or fresh garlic juice; both are antibacterial agents and will speed the healing of blemishes. If you're prone to more frequent outbreaks, try this daily treatment: Clean your face with a yogurt and honey wash (add a few tablespoons of organic honey to a cup of natural yogurt); honey is a gentle cleanser and skin conditioner, and yogurt helps smooth the skin as it cleans and exfoliates.

Blackheads, those blocked pores that often appear on the nose, chin, and forehead, can be tough to get rid of, and dermatologists agree that it's best to avoid trying to do so by squeezing. To help unclog blocked pores without damaging your skin, try a refreshing peppermint steam: Combine a handful of fresh peppermint leaves, two table-spoons of dried peppermint, and a few drops of peppermint oil. Place in a pan of boiling water. Drape a towel over your head, and let the steam bathe your face for a few minutes; the steam will unblock your pores. Next, gently rub your face with the inside of a fresh papaya skin; this will slough away old, dead skin cells, while condition-ing your skin with vitamins A and C. A faster and also effective blackhead treatment is to mix honey with equal parts of rolled oats and almond meal; the combination acts to draw out oil and dirt from your pores while exfoliating.

SHAVING SOOTHER

Removing hair from under the armpits is an unhealthy procedure since it requires close con-tact with vulnerable lymph nodes that can easily become contaminated. However, many women do remove their leg hair. Often, when a razor is used, the skin becomes irritated. The best advice is to use a loofah or other natural exfoliator *before* you shave to remove dead skin and to en-courage hairs to grow out, not in. Follow with a moisturizer of pure aloe vera, which has both soothing and healing properties.

VARICOSE VEIN TREATMENT

Unfortunately, there's no natural beauty secret that will eliminate varicose veins. This is an inherited condition that requires surgery for removal. However, there is a treatment that can help relieve the swelling and ease the discomfort of enlarged blood vessels: Lie with your legs elevated, and apply a compress of apple cider vinegar to the veiny areas; then massage the problem spots. Cider vinegar has an astringent quality that may help shrink the distended veins. In addition, avoid standing for long periods of time, and incorporate exercise routines that don't tax the legs, such as cycling and swimming; avoid aerobics, running, and bicycling.

SUN SPOT REMOVER

If you have visible sun damage (spots or freckles), you might want to try dabbing the area daily with fresh lemon juice, which acts as a bleach. Some people find the lemon too acidic and have had irritating reactions. If this is the case for you, discontinue use. Always follow with a natural moisturizer.

LIP HEALER

If your lips get chapped, you can find relief by making your own balm. Simply melt a dollop of beeswax in a double boiler with two teaspoons of almond oil. Stir well, cook, cool, and apply to your lips. This balm can be safely stored in a tight container for a day or two.

NATURAL LIP COLOR

Mashed berries combined with a bit of petroleum jelly or aloe vera make an attractive lip stain. Many commercial lipsticks, when used regularly, can drain the lips of their natural color.

After a home spa session, you're cleansed and relaxed. The emotional toll of the day is washed away; you're surrounded by a golden light. Take advantage of your good mood to embrace your loved ones and share the joy.

7

A Guide to Natural, Nutritional Purifiers

*The natural healing force within
each one of us is the greatest
force in getting well. Our food
should be our medicine. Our
medicine should be our food.*
—Hippocrates

When I was younger, I was more concerned with keeping my weight down than with what I was putting into my body. Diet sodas, weight-loss drinks, nonfattening and low-calorie foods packed with artificial ingredients and preservatives were my staples. As a result of this nonnutritional diet, my body was always in crisis. I was the first to catch seasonal colds and flus; I suffered with chronic headaches, fatigue, and fuzzy thoughts. My complexion was uneven, my teeth were decaying, and my hair and nails were brittle and dull.

A decade later I've turned all this damage around, thanks to detoxing fasts, exercise, sauna programs, and a vigilantly healthy diet that includes herbs, vitamins, and specific foods for specific cleansings. Through experience, I'm convinced that the food I eat today is truly my body of tomorrow.

This reference chapter is broken down into four sections: "Power Foods," "Healing Herbs," "Vital Vitamins," and "Mighty Minerals." Keep the guide handy so that when you plan your meals, you can incorporate its information. Pay attention to what your body is telling you. As you become more sensitive, you'll intuitively know what specific foods your body is craving, what herbs it needs, and which vitamin regimen is best for you.

POWER FOODS

NOTE: Whenever you can, plant and grow or purchase and prepare foods that are organic and in season.

Apple Pectin. This eliminates all toxins from the system. Drink apple teas; use as a sweetener; add to soups, salads, and casseroles. Apple pectin can also be taken in capsule form. Any way you get it into the system on a daily basis is a great help in purifying the body of daily exposure to pollutants and chemicals.

Asparagus. From earliest times this vegetable was used for its medicinal properties. For spring detox fasts, asparagus is highly valued for its diuretic qualities as well as for its high mineral and rutin content.

Banana. When your tummy's uneasy, skip the antacids and grab a banana. A study at the Institute of Medicine in Delhi, India, found that this fruit settles the stomach just as well as medicine. The primary reason for its beneficial effect is that bananas are high in potassium, which neutralizes stomach acid. They also spur the secretion of mucus, which coats the stomach, easing discomfort.

Beans. Beans were already a tradition as one of the Three Sisters of Life among Native Americans when the Europeans arrived. Today we know that the protein content of dried beans combines well with that of whole grains and can form the base of a nutritious vegetarian meal. Much higher in nitrogen-rich protein than grains, a healthy portion of beans is 1:4 to 1:3 that of grains.

CAUTION: Too much protein can put stress on liver and kidneys.

Broccoli. This vegetable is part of the family of so-called cruciferous vegetables. Chemicals known as indoles and isothiocynates, which are found in cruciferous vegetables, are thought to help prevent cell damage and possibly head off cancer. In addition, broccoli is a good source of vitamins A and C, and it contains five grams of protein per one-cup serving. However, it is best to note that broccoli, and cauliflower, are best *never eaten raw*. Both contain a toxin against their predators that is dispelled through heating.

Brussels Sprout. Besides containing significant amounts of the antioxidant viamins A and C, brussels sprouts contain a little-understood chemical called sulfuraphane. Recent research suggests that this chemical could be the main reason why people who eat brussels sprouts have considerably less risk of developing a wide range of cancers than those who don't. For the best benefits, it's preferable to eat brussels sprouts raw. But if that taste is intolerable, cook them lightly.

Cabbage. High in fiber and anticancer chemicals, cabbage also provides vitamin C and potassium. To tame its gas-producing effect, parboil it for five minutes, throw the cooking water out, rinse it, and then resume cooking with fresh water.

Carrot. If your mother told you that carrots were good for your eyes, she was right. Carrots are a good source of vitamin A, which is important to vision. What's more, carrots are among the richest sources of beta-carotene. In studies conducted by the U.S. Department of Agriculture, volunteers who ate two to three carrots a day saw their cholesterol levels fall an average of 11 percent. The key to preparing this healthy root is to scrub it with a stiff brush just before use. Rarely does the carrot need paring; valuable minerals lie just beneath its surface. The admonition to chew well applies to eating carrot sticks; otherwise their goodness can pass right through the digestive tract, mostly as bulk.

Cauliflower. Like broccoli, cauliflower should never be eaten raw. However, when blanched and served fresh and slightly cooked, it is ideal for relieving the pain of arthritis, and its natural sodium content is said to help excrete troublesome acid.

Corn. This vegetable gets its color from an antioxidant called lutein, which plays a special role in preventing macular degeneration, one of the leading causes of blindness among older people. Lutein and its chemical cousin zeaxanthin are found just behind the iris, where their color helps protect the retina from potentially damaging light rays. A diet rich in both (including not only corn but also dark green vegetables like spinach) may significantly lower the risk of macular degeneration.

Cranberry. Recent studies show that the cranberry contains a chemical that helps block bacteria that can cause urinary tract infections. Cranberry juice is also effective against urinary tract infections.

Cucumber. Long noted for improving the complexion, cleansing the liver, and aiding in digestion, diabetes, and headaches, cucumbers help us keep "cool" as one of them in summer months.

Fennel. Related to the carrot and resembling celery, fennel combines the sweetness of one with the juicy crispness of the other, while being more delicate than either. In ancient Greece fennel was planted in the temple garden to honor the gods; worshipers crowned their heads with airy fronds. The aromatic essential oil characteristic in fennel permeates the plant with qualities that aid digestion, stimulate glandular secretions, and help eyesight. The oil concentrates in the seeds, which are familiar to us as seasoning and as an herb tea.

Fiber. There are two kind of fiber: soluble (in water) and insoluble. Most fiber foods have both kinds, but insoluble predominates, doing its work in the intestines. Fiber makes up the bulk of the stalks, skins, peels, husks of produce and whole grains. The body can't digest it well, so it passes right through, carrying potential cancer-causing substances and at the same time making you regular and preventing hemorrhoids and diverticular disease. Soluble fiber is more digestible and works mostly in the stomach. It's the main type of fiber in oranges, strawberries, melons, and root vegetables: whole grains, beans, and peas also have large amounts. This is the fiber that makes you feel full quite quickly, so it's helpful for weight loss and weight control. This is also the cholesterol-fighting fiber. Farther down in the intestines, oat bran, in particular, can envelop molecules of cholesterol. What's more, soluble fiber slows down the body's absorption of sugar, keeping both sugar cravings in check and helping control diabetes.

Fish. Fish contains a beneficial form of fat called omega-3. It comes in two forms: eicosapentaenoic (EPA) and docosahexaenoic acid (DHA). These are actually created by an undersea vegetation that is eaten by the fish. Accumulated amounts of EPA and DHA help reduce the level of "bad" cholesterol—low-density lipoprotein or LDL—which sharply reduces the risk of atherosclerosis (hardening of the arteries). Omega-3s are also thought to help lower blood pressure. In laboratory animals, omega-3s have been found to slow the growth in the brain of amyloid protein deposits, which are characteristic of Alzheimer's disease. Researchers are also intrigued that Eskimos get 40 percent of their calories from fat, a huge portion of that fat being omega-3s, yet almost never get breast or colon cancer. Tests on laboratory animals have shown that omega-3s actually block the growth of cancers of the breast, prostate, pancreas, and colon. No one knows how this works, and the results haven't been duplicated in humans, but it's thought that the omega-3s inhibit the body's production of hormonelike substances called prostaglandins that can stimulate tumor growth. And omega-3s can actually hold back the kind of overactive immune system that produces such autoimmune diseases as rheumatoid arthritis and psoriasis.

However, be aware that fish may contain high levels of mercury and other pollutants. As a rule small fish contain lower levels of potential carcinogens.

Hardy Greens. All members of the chicory family—escarole, radicchio, and endive—strengthen the spleen, liver, kidneys, and other organs in their functions and are best eaten in late summer and fall since they are particularly helpful in preparing us for cold weather.

Horseradish. Horseradish (and other spicy foods like jalapeño or cayenne pepper) loosen up mucus secretions and increase blood flow in the sinuses, relieving the congestion that causes sinus headaches. Try one teaspoon to one tablespoon of freshly grated horseradish, or the same amount of commercially prepared horseradish preserved with vinegar. Add a bit of honey to taste if desired.

Kale. As the snow recedes in the northern part of the country, hearty kale that has wintered over from last season's planting appears bright and green as it leafs out for spring picking. Packed with vitamins, kale can fortify us through the vulnerability of our body's seasonal transition from cold to warmth.

Licorice. Glycyrrhizic acid and other, as yet unknown licorice compounds have been shown to be anticancer, anti-inflammatory, antiulcer, and anticavity, as well as immune-stimulating. For licorice to provide these healthful benefits, make sure to purchase real licorice root, which is most often sold in health food stores.

CAUTION: While licorice is considered safe to consume in small amounts for brief periods, check with a doctor before using it in medicinal doses.

Mushroom. The common type of mushroom sold in most supermarkets is a healthy choice. Even better, though, is the special variety of mushroom known as shitake. This mushroom has long been prized for its medicinal properties in the Orient, and recently scientists have analyzed it to discover that it contains compounds unlike those found in other plants. Shitake is especially effective as a treatment for systemic conditions related to immunity, aging, and sexual dysfunction thanks to the polysaccharide lentinan, a proved immune booster.

Onion. The onion is renowned for the cancer-fighting ability of a chemical it contains called allyl sulfide, which not only retards the spread of cancer cells but also aids the production of enzymes that help the body rid itself of substances that cause cancer. Onions have been found to have other health-promoting properties. For example, some studies show that onion extracts decrease lipid levels in the blood and lower blood pressure. According to other studies, onion consumption may also decrease the risk of heart disease. In addition, onions may have antimicrobial effects, and they can lower blood sugar levels, suggesting a possible use in the treatment of diabetes. The healing properties of the onion have long been used in treating colds, from wrapping slices in a hot cloth and applying it externally for sore throats to making a syrup of grated onion and honey to drink in hot milk or cider as a remedy for coughing. Onions also offer potassium, fiber, and some protein.

Orange. This ancient fruit has been cultivated for more than four thousand years and is known for its vitamin C content. In addition, studies from the U.S. Department of Agriculture suggest that oranges may stop the development of cataracts.

Parsnip. This sweetmeat of the root vegetable family can be used in numerous recipes, even in desserts fit for a diabetic diet. Not only are parsnips naturally sweet, but they contain inulin, a substance similar to insulin. High in minerals, parsnips enrich our winter fare, warm us from the inside out, can strengthen weak stomachs, and in olden times were the dietary choice for those with TB or a fever.

Radish. Most people enjoy rinsing the radish and dipping it in salt. But beware that too much salt can cause the radish to feel like lead in your stomach. Otherwise radishes are an excellent aid to digestion. They are also valued highly for those with liver or gallbladder problems. More recently, radishes have been found to be helpful against skin eruptions, herpes, acne, and boils.

Rhubarb. Remarkably rich in vitamins A and C and minerals, rhubarb revitalizes the blood, brings digestion to order, and sparks lackluster appetites.

Soy Foods. Soybeans, tofu, miso, tempeh, soy milk, and soy cheese contain isoflavines and other chemicals that may block the action of estrogen in the body, helping prevent the development of breast and ovarian cancers as well as hot flashes and other menopausal symptoms. Soy protein may also reduce the risk of osteoporosis by helping the body retain more calcium. In addition, a recent study reported that soy protein can help reduce blood cholesterol levels; substitute a soy protein source for at least half your protein intake.

Spinach. Originating as a wild vegetable in the Caucasian area of the Middle East, spinach was brought to Europe in the sixteenth century. Cultivated widely since then, it has been recognized as high in chlorophyll, vitamins, and minerals.

CAUTION: Select only organically grown spinach, because chemical fertilizers tend to produce leaves containing high levels of nitrates. Spinach also should not be subjected to heat for more than a few minutes, only until bright green in color, and should never be reheated. Long cooking develops its oxalic acid content into an intolerable form that is best avoided.

Tea. Green tea and its fermented version, black tea (regular or decaf), are truly healthful tonics, brimming with versatile antioxidant compounds that have the same antiaging and anticancer effects as vitamin E and C but are much more powerful. Chinese studies showed that rates of esophageal cancer were 20 percent lower in men and 50 percent in women who drank at least one cup of tea a day. Tea also helps prevent the blood clots that trigger stroke and heart attack. Researchers in Holland found that men who drank just a few cups per day had one-third the rate of fatal heart disease of those who drank less. As little as one cup per day lowers blood pressure. Other benefits include its tranquilizing effects and reduction in tooth decay, thanks to the tannins that weaken bacteria.

Tomato. The pigment that saturates the tomato with color is called lycopene, and according to research, it is one of the strongest antioxidants in the food chain. Tomatoes supply as much as 90 percent of all the lycopene many of us get; that may explain why a diet abundant in them seems to protect against several types of cancer. Researchers at the Aviano Cancer Center in Italy found that people who ate raw tomatoes at least seven times a week cut their risk of stomach, bladder, and colon cancers by half.

Vanilla. This is a natural appetite suppressant. In studies of obese people, participants ate 50 percent less after popping open a vanilla bean and inhaling deeply. Vanilla's strong aroma appears to stimulate the appetite center of the brain, tricking it into thinking it's already full.

Walnut. Adding walnuts to a low cholesterol diet can help raise levels of "good" HDL cholesterol and lower "bad" LDL cholesterol.

CAUTION: Since walnuts are also high in fat, go easy on them. One ounce of chopped black walnuts contains 170 calories and sixteen grams of fat.

Whole Grains, Brown Rice, and Oats. Recent research has shown that increased levels of the brain chemical serotonin can boost one's mood. While certain drugs can increase the level of serotonin, the right food choices can also do the job, without the potential side effects of medication. According to Dr. Joel Robertson, author of *Peak Performance Living,* adding complex carbohydrates—particularly whole grains, brown rice, and oats—to your diet can help alleviate depression by increasing serotonin levels.

Yam. Some of the unpleasant symptoms of menopause can be avoided by putting a few yams into the weekly diet. Menopausal flushes and chills are the body's response to the sudden decrease in estrogen production; yams contain a natural form of estrogen that can help alleviate discomfort.

Yarrow Tea. Purifies the liver.

Yogurt. Live cultures found in yogurt, such as as *Lactobacillus acidophilus,* can relieve intestinal discomfort caused by mild food poisoning. For those on antibiotics, yogurt can relieve the diarrhea that often results from an overgrowth of bacteria normally present in the colon. Eating yogurt may also help prevent yeast infections, but not all yogurts contain live and active cultures; check ingredient lists.

HEALING HERBS

Allspice. Renowned for aiding digestion and relieving pain, allspice is an herb from the Caribbean that has the flavors of cinnamon, pepper, juniper, and clove. The chemical eugenol is believed to be the source of this herb's healing power. Eugenol, which is also found in clove, may help the action of the enzymes needed for digestion. It relieves pain and is used in some commercial remedies for toothache.

Aloe. Use aloe to heal minor cuts and burns. Simply applying the clear gel that oozes out of a cut leaf can speed the healing of a minor wound. In addition, aloe may slow the growth of bacteria, preventing the infection of wounds.

Barberry. Said to have been used in ancient Egypt to fight off the plague, barberry today is known for its antibiotic effect. Its active ingredient is berberine, which sets the body's white blood cells in action against a wide variety of infections. There are a host of other conditions that barberry is said to treat. In Europe, for example, it is the traditional remedy for pinkeye, and in Russia it is used to treat high blood pressure. Experts speculate that barberry dilates blood vessels.

CAUTION: This herb is dangerous in high doses and should not be taken by anyone with a chronic illness.

Basil. Long used as a spice in cooking, basil originated in India, and references to it are found in the Bible. Basil has shown itself to be an effective treatment for acne and intestinal parasites, and as an immune stimulant. For these purposes, basil oil is usually used, since it is more concentrated than other extracts of the herb.

CAUTION: Basil may have estrogenlike effects and should not be used by pregnant or nursing women.

Bilberry. This herb is most effective in tincture form. The active principles in bilberry are known for its hypoglycemic agents. It is indicated for fatigue and symptoms associated with hypoglycemia, diabetes, and elevated cholesterol.

Burdock Root. Rich in flavonoids, ligans, and bitter glycosides, burdock root has an insulin content of up to 45 percent, making it valuable in treating diabetes. Its high levels of lignans and inulin have proven anti-inflammatory effects, which explain its use in such conditions as acute laryngitis and skin inflammation. Burdock also has a long history of use as a detoxifier in skin conditons. In *Herbal Medications* herbalists A. W. and L. R. Priest write that burdock "influences skin, kidneys, mucous and serous membranes to remove accumulated waste products. It is specifically beneficial in healing eruptions on the head, face and neck, and for acute irritable and inflammatory conditions." It can be used for eczema, psoriasis, boils, and similar skin toxicity conditions. Taken in tea form, burdock makes an excellent cleanser.

Calendula. I used a cream based on this versatile herb to protect my son from diaper rash when he was an infant. It is often used in oils for massage, in baths for inflammatory skin problems, and in tinctures for ulcers and digestive problems. It can be used topically as an antiseptic and for ulcers and varicose veins, as well as orally against parasites.

Caraway. Although caraway seeds are used to flavor rye bread, they are also an effective remedy for digestive ills. For instance, the chemical carvol and carvene in the seeds have been found to calm the muscle tissue of the digestive system. This antispasmodic action may also help relax the uterus, easing menstrual cramps.

CAUTION: Caraway taken as an herbal supplement can be dangerous for pregnant or nursing women.

Chamomile. Used as an herbal remedy, chamomile relieves insomnia, nervousness, upset stomach, and menstrual cramps. At least some studies have found that chamomile contains substances that may help ease cramping and inflammation.

CAUTION: Although reactions to chamomile are extremely rare, it is possible to have an allergic reaction since chamomile tea contains pollen.

Cinnamon. This herb has a reputation as an antiseptic and pain reliever. Surprisingly, it is able to kill bacteria, fungi, and viruses. Some people even use it on minor cuts to help prevent infection. Since cinnamon contains eugenol (see allspice above), an oil that is a natural pain reliever, it is sometimes used to relieve the sting of minor cuts. Finally, cinnamon may increase the action of digestive enzymes, aiding digestion.

Dandelion. Bloating, constipation, indigestion, colds, and congestive heart failure respond to the dandelion. According to clinical studies, dandelion root aids the flow of bile and helps improve such conditions as liver congestion, bile duct inflammation, gallstones, and jaundice. The plant also seems to stimulate the appetite and helps digestion.

Echinacea. Commonly known as coneflower, echinacea was first used by Native Americans to treat both illnesses and injuries. Now it has a reputation for preventing or treating colds and upper respiratory infections. Studies in Europe have shown that this herb stimulates the immune system and appears to ease the symptoms of colds as well as to lessen the time between infections. The herb comes in several types of preparations, but the liquid extract (usually in alcohol) appears to work best.

Feverfew. The herb feverfew is used mainly in the prevention and treatment of migraines and the treatment of inflammation and fever. In treating migraines, it has been shown to reduce both the number and the severity of attacks. Feverfew may stop the production of chemicals in the body that promote inflammation, thereby easing the pain of arthritis.

NOTE: If you have a blood clotting disorder, consult your physician before taking this herb.

Garlic. Certain sulfur-based compounds in garlic may prevent the spread of breast and prostate cancers; they also inhibit colon, esophageal, and skin cancers—in some cases by killing cancer cells outright. Garlic compounds thin the blood, preventing clotting and lowering cholesterol and blood pressure. In lab cultures, its compounds improve memory and learning in aged mice, lending credibility to garlic's ancient use as a prescription for senile dementia in China. In addition, garlic stimulates the release of the brain's natural tranquilizer, serotonin. Two to three cloves of raw garlic a day will also help lower cholesterol levels. Aged garlic powder or extract in pills contains concentrated amounts of garlic's active chemicals.

What's more, if you have a wart and want to try a home remedy that has been known to work, crush a garlic clove and place enough on the wart to cover it. Bandage and keep the wart covered for twenty-four hours. The blister that should form will take approximately one week to fall off.

Ginger. First used medicinally in China, ginger is now known for its action against motion sickness, indigestion, and nausea. In fact, studies have shown that ginger is more effective than the over-the-counter drug Dramamine in combating motion sickness as well as effective against morning sickness. Since this herb can also slow the formation of prostaglandins (hormonelike substances), when given to patients with rheumatoid arthritis, it has increased mobility and decreased stiffness, swelling, and pain. This proven blood thinner has been shown to be at least as effective as some prescription drugs in blocking the production of thromboxane, which makes blood platelets stick together. Ginger comes in several forms, including dry powdered root, tea, and fresh ginger. The dry root is more effective than the tea form.

CAUTION: Ginger is generally considered safe, though taking more than six grams on an empty stomach may cause some irritation of the stomach lining.

Gingko. This herb has the therapeutic action for circulatory problems related to arteriosclerosis, memory loss, vertigo, and hearing loss. Test trials with oral dosing of gingko extract have shown neurotransmitter-modulating activity, accounting for gingko's ability to improve concentration.

Ginseng. This best known of the traditional Chinese herbal remedies has the power to revitalize. In studies with mice, ginseng helped slow the onset of exhaustion; research in humans has shown that it has the ability to improve both physical and mental performance.

CAUTION: Ginseng should be used with caution. It can be toxic if overused; side effects include high blood pressure and hot flashes.

Hawthorn Berry. Taken in tincture form, hawthorn improves cardiac muscle contractibility and is especially recommended to fortify the heart muscle and the coronary vessel. This herb is a useful remedy for stress from overwork and from the natural results of aging.

Lavender. The essential oil that sparked the current interest in aromatherapy, lavender is widely used externally for its mild pain-relieving and anti-inflammatory effects. It is a favorite first-aid remedy for not only burns but also minor wounds, sprains, insect bites and stings, athlete's foot, and muscular aches and pains. Lavender's fresh, flowery aroma has a sedating effect and can help induce sleep, alleviate stress, and reduce depression and nervous tension. You can buy it as a concentrated liquid and in a variety of body care products.

Milk Thistle. Indicated for digestive disturbances especially caused by liver complaints, bloating, and high-fat–high-cholesterol diets, milk thistle is a useful treatment for jaundice, cirrhosis of the liver, and intoxication.

Mullein. The leaves of mullein have been used for hundreds of years in Ayurvedic, Native American, and European herbalism for the treatment of colds, coughs, sore throats, and bronchitis. The velvety leaves are rich in mucilage, a gelatinous substance that soothes irritated mucous membranes and bronchial passages. Although sipping mullein tea can be very effective, expect a bitter taste; either brew it with sweet marshmallow root or add a dollop of honey to improve its flavor.

Oregano. This herb is a natural cold reliever. The chemicals carvacrol and thymol in oregano act as expectorants, loosening secretions in the lungs. A weak oregano tea is often enough to soothe the coughs and congestions of colds and flus. In addition, oregano helps digestion by relaxing the muscles of the digestive tract.

Parsley. Thriving since antiquity, parsley is the most popular of all herbaceous plants. Rich in potassium, it aids digestion. It also possesses high concentrations of vitamins and minerals. Parsley promotes blood circulation as well as strengthens the kidneys and nervous system.

Sarsaparilla Root. This herb provides the characteristic taste of root beer and has a history of use in Europe as a blood purifier dating back to the sixteenth century. Several saponin ingredients in sarsaparilla have been shown to be effective in treating psoriasis. In a controlled study one of these components, sarsaponin, greatly improved psoriasis in 62 percent of the patients and completely cleared the disease in 18 percent, according to the *New England Journal of Medicine*. Sarsaparilla binds endotoxins, which are cell wall constituents of bacteria that are absorbed from the digestive tract. If these endotoxins are allowed to bypass the liver and circulate in the blood, they contribute to gout, arthritis, and psoriasis. Three to twelve grams of dried sarsaparilla root per day as a tea or in capsule form are recommended.

Tumeric. This spice, used in Indian cooking to impart a deep golden color to curries, also has powerful antiseptic properties and is lethal to any form of bacterium. A combination of ghee, tumeric, and finely chopped onions makes an excellent poultice to help drain boils and kill bacteria. Consult a physician before treating boils in the region of the groin or armpit. Infections in these areas can easily be picked up by the lymphatic system and spread throughout the body. Also be aware that tumeric will stain anything it touches.

Valerian. This herb is indicated for the relief of nervousness and insomnia. Low doses taken during the day can help stabilize the nervous system so as to induce normal sleep patterns. Numerous scientific studies have confirmed valerian's relaxant effects, and several studies have found that it is as effective as some barbiturates for reducing the time needed to fall asleep. Valerian can also be used as an antispasmodic to relieve back spasms.

VITAL VITAMINS

If you maintain an *ideal* diet with plenty of fresh, organic vegetables, whole grains, and nourishing protein, then you won't need to take any vitamin supplements other than a daily mineral-fortified multiple vitamin. Personally I have reservations about consuming large doses of supplements. Vitamins can have side effects, especially when taken in megadoses. If you suffer from a medical condition or illness, if you take any medication, or if you are pregnant or nursing, consult your physician before taking vitamins.

This said, there have been numerous scientific studies supporting the beneficial effects of added doses of vitamins, especially when targeting specific conditions.

Vitamin A (carotenoids, beta-carotene, retinol). This fat-soluble vitamin is important to vision, skin, teeth, bones, and mucous membranes. For instance, vitamin A is essential to the production of pigments that help you see in low light. A deficiency of vitamin A can result in night blindness. Furthermore, by helping keep the skin and mucous membranes healthy (Retin-A is a vitamin A–based prescription cream that reduces the skin's visible signs of aging), vitamin A helps the body fight infections. Finally, vitamin A—especially in its preliminary form as a carotenoid—is an antioxidant.

RDA*: 5,000 IU† for men; 4,000 IU for women. Food sources: sweet potato, pumpkin, spinach, carrot.

CAUTION: In high doses, vitamin A is toxic. Beta-carotene is generally not considered toxic.

Vitamin C (ascorbic acid, sodium ascorbate). Vitamin C's best-known health effect is its reputation for curing the common cold. Although the vitamin appears to have some antihistamine effects, there are no studies that demonstrate that it can actually prevent colds. However, vitamin C does have many health effects as an antioxidant. For example, it may protect against heart disease;

* Recommended daily amount.
† International unit.

studies show that people with the highest risk of heart disease also have the lowest blood levels of C. It may also help prevent the formation of blood clots, offering protection against heart attack and stroke. Even low blood pressure has been linked to high levels of vitamin C.

RDA: 60 milligrams.
Food sources: fresh fruits (especially oranges and cantaloupe) and vegetables.

CAUTION: Megadoses can cause diarrhea and, in some people, kidney stones. Large doses may interfere with copper absorption; chewable C can erode the enamel on teeth.

Vitamin D (cholecalciferol). Made by the skin when exposed to sunlight, vitamin D aids in the absorption of calcium and phosphorus, thus helping maintain strong bones and teeth. By so doing, vitamin D may reduce the risk of osteoporosis, a thinning of the bones.

RDA: 5 micrograms of 200 IU.
Food sources: Although vitamin D is found in fortified milk, butter, eggs and yogurt, I prefer to steer clear of dairy products. Instead, get your vitamin D from fish (like tuna) and fortified cereals.

CAUTION: An excess of vitamin D can be toxic. If an overdose leads to elevated blood levels of calcium, the result can do permanent damage to the kidneys, heart, and other organs.

Vitamin E (tocopherol, alpha-tocopherol). This vitamin makes an important contribution to any antiaging and detoxing treatment. It's been shown that vitamin E can slow down the damage caused by free radicals in the body, thereby protecting tissues of the brain, eyes, lungs, kidneys, and liver from age-related changes. Some studies suggest that E may prevent or delay the damage of Parkinson's disease and other age-related illnesses. In addition, one of E's most potent effects is its ability to deter clots by preventing cholesterol from blocking arteries. Some researchers believe that this property of vitamin E means it protects against heart attacks.

RDA: 10 milligrams for men; 8 milligrams for women.
Food sources: wheat germ oil, hazelnuts, sunflower seeds, and sunflower oil.
CAUTION: Vitamin E appears to be safe at dosages of 400 IU daily. But because it may affect blood clotting, consult your physician before taking supplements over the RDA.

Folic Acid (folate or folacin). This B vitamin plays a role in the formation of DNA and RNA, in growth, and in the metabolism of protein. Too little folic acid may raise your odds of colon, lung, or cervical cancer. In a Harvard study those who ate the most folic acid were a third less apt to have polyps that can lead to colon cancer than those who ate the least folic acid. Low folic acid levels also have been linked to serious depression, dementia, memory loss, and low mental acuity, even in the young. In addition, adequate folic acid intake could prevent three thousand neural tube birth defects every year, according to the Centers for Disease Control and Prevention.

RDA: 400 micrograms; for those over fifty, 500 micrograms.
Food sources: It's tough to get enough folic acid in food because the vitamin is poorly absorbed. So it makes sense not only to eat foods rich in folic acid like brewer's yeast, asparagus, brussels sprouts, and avocado but to take supplements as well.

Vitamin B$_6$ (pyridoxine). B$_6$ has been shown to be effective in improving PMS symptoms, including depression, irritability, breast pain, and bloating. New research shows that it also soothes some of the symptoms of carpal tunnel syndrome, a condition caused by repetitive hand motions.

RDA: 2 milligrams for men; 1.6 milligrams for women.

Food sources: bananas, chicken, halibut, boiled potatoes.

CAUTION: Vitamin B_6 is one of the few water-soluble vitamins that have the potential for toxicity. High doses can cause numbness and neurological disorders.

MIGHTY MINERALS

Boron. Most people connect boron with 20-Mule Team borax and reruns of *Death Valley Days,* but evidence is mounting of this trace mineral's importance in maintaining youthful bones and preventing osteoporosis. Boron is involved with the body's use of bone-building vitamin D, calcium, and phosphorus, and it seems to keep bones from losing calcium and other minerals.

RDA: 1 to 2 milligrams a day, obtainable in food.

Food sources: Almonds, dates, hazelnuts, honey, peanuts, prunes, raisins.

Calcium. A must for strong bones, calcium is especially important for the average woman. Optimal calcium intake before age twenty-five is crucial for building bones that are resistant to osteoporosis. It has also been shown to reduce the risk of colon cancer, heart disease, and high blood pressure.

RDA: 800 milligrams for adults over age twenty-five; for ages eleven to twenty-five, and pregnant and breast-feeding women, 1,200 milligrams.

Food sources: dairy products, such as milk and cheese, as well as beans and peas and such vegetables as broccoli, spinach, kale, and chard. There is some debate about the amount of calcium that is actually available in vegetables since vegetables contain oxalic acid. When this enzyme is combined with calcium, the body may be prevented from absorbing calcium. On the other hand, citric acid can increase calcium's absorption.

CAUTION: Large doses may contribute to the formation of kidney stones.

Chromium. There's been a lot of hype around chromium as a weight-loss aid, but recently the FDA has cracked down on some of the more fantastic claims. The truth is that this trace mineral is essential to help your body's insulin regulate blood sugar levels; if your body's blood sugar regulation is just partly out of whack, you may be faced with constant sugar cravings and an increased calorie intake. All degrees of impairment can be called glucose intolerance, and chromium deficiency is considered the number one cause. Nutritionists say that most of us have at least borderline deficiencies of chromium. The main cause of these deficiencies is our large consumption of refined grains and sugar. These foods dump huge amounts of carbohydrates into the system, and the chromium that occurs naturally in whole grains is often removed in processing. The youth factor also comes into play: As we age, our bodies can't store as much chromium, and if we don't get enough in our diets, we can develop deficiencies and even diabetes or hypoglycemia. Chromium also lowers LDL cholesterol.

RDA: Not yet established, but adults should get from 50 to 200 micrograms daily.
Food sources: brewer's yeast, whole grains, potatoes with skin.

CAUTION: Generally, chromium supplements are considered safe since the body accepts only 2 to 10 percent of what is ingested. However, because chromium supplements can change the need for insulin, people with diabetes should not take chromium supplements without their doctors' permission.

Iron. This is an essential ingredient for a tough immune system, and the body needs it to make antibodies. Stress, menstruation, heavy exercise, or a vegetarian diet can drain iron from the body, preventing the manufacture of hemoglobin, the substance in red blood cells that carries oxygen to all parts of the body. Lack of hemoglobin can cause anemia, exhaustion, difficulty concentrating, and loss of appetite—all problems that make you feel and look old.

RDA: for men 10 milligrams; for women 15 milligrams. Pregnant women need 30 milligrams. If you eat a balanced whole foods diet, you should have no problem getting enough iron. Still, research shows that 57 percent of Americans don't get enough iron in their diets.
Food sources: red meat (to be avoided, generally), free-range poultry, green vegetables, nuts, cast-iron cookware, fortified cereals. Vitamin C can help the body absorb iron from nonmeat sources. Be aware that calcium and caffeine inhibit iron absorption.

CAUTION: Too much iron can be dangerous; it's a strong risk factor for heart disease. Do not overdose with supplements.

Magnesium. This trace mineral is part of bones and teeth. It's also necessary for the manufacture of proteins, for the relaxation of muscles, for the release of energy, and for many metabolic reactions. Magnesium helps control calcium levels in the blood by aiding the function of the parathyroid hormone. If you crave chocolate, you might want to try magnesium instead. This mineral may curb such cravings, especially for women during their monthly cycles. It also reduces the risk of toxemia during pregnancy, prevents osteoporosis, and boosts mood and energy levels, particularly in women suffering from fatigue caused by stress. Other studies have shown magnesium may play a role in controlling blood pressure.

RDA: 350 milligrams for men; 280 milligrams for women.
Food sources: green leafy vegetables, dairy products, peas, beans, and nuts.

Potassium. It helps the body maintain its water balance, and it is also involved in transmitting messages between nerves and between nerves and muscles. In addition, this mineral is necessary for the metabolism of carbohydrates and proteins. A diet rich in potassium may help keep blood pressure low and reduce the risk of having a stroke. One long-term study found that subjects who ate the least amount of potassium had a greater risk of dying from a stroke. For men, the risk was two and a half times greater; for women, it was five times greater.

RDA: none; generally an intake between 2,000 and 3,000 milligrams recommended for adults.
Food sources: fruits (bananas and cantaloupe are especially high), dairy products, beans, and peas.

Selenium. Another antioxidant in the body's free radical fighting arsenal, this mineral plays a crucial role in making sure the immune system is in full force. In addition, selenium intake has been linked to a reduced risk of cancer. One study, for example, found that people with low blood levels of selenium had the highest risk for cancer: six times more than people with high levels of selenium. Selenium may prompt the liver to detoxify chemicals.

RDA: 70 micrograms for men; 55 micrograms for women.
Food sources: meats, fish, and some grains. The average American diet usually meets the RDA without the need for supplements.
    CAUTION: Large doses can be poisonous since the detoxifying process spurred by selenium can cause the release of carcinogens.

Zinc. This mineral is crucial for a smooth-running effective immune system. Poor wound healing is one of the early symptoms of low zinc levels. Adequate zinc reduces the risk of heart disease and slows bone loss. Low levels of zinc may contribute to a tendency to suffer from infections and related diseases.

RDA: 15 milligrams for men; 12 milligrams for women.

Food sources: meat, poultry, eggs, whole grains, and oysters. If you intend to get your zinc from whole grains, get it in the form of whole grain bread. Whole grains contain a substance that prevents the absorption of zinc, but yeast blocks the action of the substance.

CAUTION: Large doses can cause diarrhea, fever, kidney failure, and, in some extreme cases, death.

8

Afterword: Renewal and Celebration

God bless the roots! Body and soul are one!
—Theodore Roethke

Our bodies are composed of the four essential elements: earth, water, air, and fire. Every earthly organism comprises these four elements, and each element has its correspondent in the universe. Since what composes the body (microcosm) also makes up the universe (macrocosm), we need to create a deep harmony between the two. If your detox was successful, you've experienced this harmony; you are enjoying the balance between a healthy body and a healthy mind because sickness is nothing but imbalance. Where there is harmony, there is also health.

Do not doubt that the mind is powerful. There

was a time when I expended a lot of negative energy judging myself by other people's standards, and as a result, I often engendered feelings of insecurity. Somehow I hadn't learned that I would never find peace as long as I worried about what other people thought of me. But as I got closer to understanding the importance of purifying my thoughts along with my body, I began to ask myself why I bothered. Why couldn't I let go and give others the liberty to think what they will?

This is the basis for the art of pure living: Negativity hurts only those who think negatively of themselves. In reality we are damaged only by our own toxic opinion of ourselves. The whole problem of insecurity and feelings of inadequacy actually comes from within, and the only way to heal this inner wound is not to think ill of ourselves—even for a moment. *No guilt.* This is one of the secrets of harmony and balance.

Another secret to living smoothly is to enjoy whatever life brings. Each moment of life, even the most trying, can turn to joy when you do this. Don't waste a precious moment worrying about the future or embracing regrets. Choose, instead, to start unfolding your infinite potential within. Never forget that the whole universe belongs to you and you are a part of the universe.

Detoxing is a wonderful way to cleanse your mind of negative distractions and to get to the heart of life's lessons. It's the surest route to turn inward, eliminating toxic thought and listening to the truth of your heart. I've heard from many people who have followed my detox program, and often they report an increase in self-confidence. This feeling is reflected in their relationships with family, friends, and coworkers. Belinda, a thirty-three-year-old graphic designer, told me that before detoxing she suffered with spells of depression, often around her menstrual cycle. "I felt hopeless," she explained. "My work and marriage were unbearable, and I would go around for days unable to appreciate my life in any real way. It felt like pure, joyless drudgery."

No wonder Belinda's world was bleak. The subtle negative energy that she emanated was communicated to the people around her. In return she received from others what she already created in herself. In other words, when you give out toxic energy, that is exactly what comes back to you.

After Belinda's detox, which included the fast and a conscientious effort to eliminate toxins from her environment and emotional life, a positivity slowly emerged. Growth, change, and optimism naturally occurred. Belinda is no longer susceptible to mood swings. Her work is satisfying and creative. She embraces her family and friends with a loving, open heart. "I feel so different. If someone told me that another soul was inhabiting my skin, I would believe them," Belinda says of her remarkable transformation. "I feel a kind of freedom I remember experiencing as a child but had lost until my detox."

If you've been living for years under a cloud of negative, life-draining energy, don't expect your reality to change completely overnight. Be easy on yourself. Although you'll feel immediate physical results from the ten-day detox, it takes time to change a lifetime of firmly rooted habits. Whenever negativity rears its head, acknowledge it, and then surround that thought with white light. Know that positive, affirmative energy is much stronger and can easily slay the fire-breathing naysayer dragon. Negative energy is not natural. It is a figment of our own creation. On the other hand, universal energy is absolute and joyous, available for you to tap into at any moment of your life.

Also, make it a habit to listen carefully to the *sound* of your words. When you have something to say, see that it comes from your heart center. To be truly heard, we must establish our connection with others by centering ourselves in love and positive energy. When you are able to speak with love, you will surely be heard, for then the heart will be speaking. When you are truly in tune with your positive center, you will be overwhelmed with friends, and you will enjoy an abundance of love. When this happens, you will know that you are finally released from the prison of judgment.

As I said before, release from negative patterns takes time. Life is a journey that continues for eternity. Be ecstatic in the knowledge that you have taken many steps toward your goal of absolute clarity and joy. If some days you fall back—negative thoughts are pervasive or you fill your diet or environment with toxic elements—don't waste energy being angry or blaming yourself. This will only add to a storehouse of negative thought. Accept yourself as an ever-evolving soul.

When we are cleansed through detoxing and can finally experience our true essence, we realize who we are. Our original nature is revealed.

Bibliography

INTRODUCTION

Paul Christian. *The History and Practice of Magic* (New York: Citadel Press, 1963), pp. 67, 107, 189.

Zolar. *The Encyclopedia of Ancient and Forbidden Knowledge* (Los Angeles: Nash Publishing, 1970), pp. 19, 271–72.

Richard Cavendish. *The Black Arts* (New York: Capricorn Books, 1967), p. 90.

BIBLIOGRAPHY

CHAPTER 1: THE TOXIC CONNECTION

Malcolm Muggeridge. Speech at Edinburgh International Festival, August 24, 1969, cited in *The Quotable Quotations Book* (New York: Crowell, 1980), p. 51.

Ingrid Zommers. "Chemical Reaction." *Natural Health,* pp. 30–32.

Diane Di Simone. "Air Raid!" *Country Living* (January 1995), pp. 10–17.

Stephen B. Edelson, M.D. Environmental and Preventative Health Center of Atlanta, Internet release, p. 1.

Wendy Deal. "Killer Outfit." *Natural Health* (August 1996), pp. 40–46.

"Cleaning the Air: Eliminate Indoor Air Pollution." *Green Living* (Winter 1995–96), pp. 22–26.

"What Are These Chemicals Doing in My Shampoo?," *Natural Health* (September–October 1996), pp. 34–35.

Kristen, McNutt, Ph.D., J.D. "Food Is Dangerous Stuff." *Nutrition Today* (March–April 1996), pp. 82–84.

Richard Laliberte. "How Safe Is Your Child's Food?" *Parents* (May 1995), pp. 30–32.

Tufts University & Nutrition News Letter (June 1996), pp. 3–5.

E. Ward. "Additives Make Food Appealing, but

Are They Safe?" *Environmental Nutrition* (July 94), pp. 6–7.

"Food That Can Kill." *Maclean's* (April 27, 1987), pp. 26–31.

Amy Rosenbaum Clark. *Vegetarian Times* (March 1995), pp. 76–80.

Elizabeth Somer, M.A., R.D. "The Scoop on MSG." *Shape* (March 1996), pp. 40–41.

Anastasia Toufexis. "The Battle Over Olestra Is Finished." *Time* (January, 1996), p. 61.

Laura Shapiro. "Fake Fat: Miracle or Menace?" *Newsweek* (January 8, 1996), pp. 60–61.

Sheila O'Connor. "Fat & Toxins." *Total Health* (December 1994), pp. 22, 44.

Marty Munson, et al. "Skipping the Fat May Save Your Sight." *Prevention* (January 1996), pp. 21–23.

Jeffrey A. Johnson, MSC, and J. Lyle Bootman, Ph.D. "Drug Related Morbidity and Mortality." Archives of Internal Medicine (October 9, 1995) pp. 1949–56.

Joseph E. Pizzorno, Jr., M.D. "Ten Drugs I Would Never Take." *Natural Health* (September–October 1996), pp. 84–85, 146–48.

Daniel Royal, D.O. "Health Hazard in Your Teeth." *Alternative Medicine Digest,* issue no. 13 (September 1996), pp. 40–43.

"Are Dental Amalgams Dangerous?" *Let's Live* (November 1996), p. 12.

BIBLIOGRAPHY

Redford Williams, M.D., and Virginia Williams, Ph.D. *Anger Kills* (New York: Times Books, 1993), pp. 45, 47.

John Carpi. "Stress . . . It's Worse Than You Think." *Psychology Today* (January–February 1996), pp. 34–41, 74–76.

United States Chamber of Commerce, 1994.

Gary Legwold. "Emotions and Your Health." *Better Homes and Gardens* (October 1994), pp. 60–61.

Williams and Williams, "Anger Kills," pp. 27–28.

Bruce Bower. "Hopelessness Tied to Heart and Cancer Deaths." *Science News* (April 13, 1996), p. 230.

"Blue Mood, Smaller Brood?" *Psychology Today* (July–August 1996), p. 16.

Gina Kolata. "Chance of Heart Attack Increases for Those Who Suffer Depression." *New York Times,* December 17, 1996, p. C-3.

Gina Kolata. "Which Comes First Depression or Heart Disease?" *New York Times,* January 14, 1997, p. C-1.

Gurudev Shree Chitrabanu. *The Psychology of Enlightenment.* (New York: Dodd Mead, 1979), pp. 7–8.

CHAPTER 2: COME CLEAN, CHANGE YOUR LIFE

Joel Fuhrman, M.D., *Fasting and Eating for Health: A Medical Doctor's Program for Conquering Disease.* (New York: St. Martin's Press, 1995).

John Baldock, compiler, *The Little Book of Zen Wisdom.* London: Element Books, 1994.

Michael Rothfeld. "Fasting: Are the Health Benefits Fact or Fiction?" In *The Detox Diet* (Elson Haas, M.D., editor). Celestial Arts, 1966.

Elson, Haas, M.D. "Get on the Fast Track." *Natural Health* (March–April 1996), pp. 50–52.

Ben Napp. "Toxic Avenger." *Fitness* (March 14, 1989), pp. 3, 7.

Roberta Wilson. "Fasting for Beauty." *Let's Live* (August 1994), pp. 62–66.

"Can You Write Your Way to Good Health?" *Psychology Today* (January–February 1997), p. 20.

"The Latest Health Barometer—Your Dreams." *First for Women* (October 10, 1996), p. 36.

Lucy Lidell. *The Sensual Body* (New York: Fireside Books, 1987), pp. 43, 50, 52, 56, 117.

Gurudev Shree Chitrabhanu, *The Psychology of Enlightenment.* (New York: Dodd Mead, 1979), pp. 3–4.

Brahma Kumaris, World Spirit Organization.

Internet:http://www.rajayoga.com

Sharon Doyle Driedger. "Prayer Power." *Maclean's* (September 25, 1995), p. 42.

CHAPTER 3: WHAT'S YOUR PERSONAL POISON?

Gurudev Shree Chitrabhanu. *The Psychology of Enlightenment.* (New York: Dodd Mead, 1979), pp. 39–40.

CHAPTER 4: READY, SET, DETOX

Trisha Thompson. "The Fasting Controversy." *Harper's Bazaar* (January 1992), pp. 80–84.

Elson M. Haas, M.D. *Staying Healthy with the Seasons* (Celestial Arts, 1981).

"2-Day Mind and Body De-tox." *First for Women* (April 1996), p. 17.

Trisha Thompson. "The Hungry High." *Harper's Bazaar* (January 1992), pp. 80–84.

Tom Deters, D.C. "Should You Fast?" *Muscle & Fitness.* (July 1995), pp. 94–95.

Ellen Albertson, R.D. "Fasting." *American Health* (July–August 1996), p. 65.

Lora B. Wilder et al., "The Effect of Fasting Status on the Determination of Low-Density and High-Density Lipoprotein Cholesterol." *American Journal of Medicine* (October 1995), pp. 374–76.

Denise Duhamel. "Holding Fast." *American Health,* pp. 44–48.

Jen Kjeldsen-Kragh et al. "Controlled Trial of Fasting and One-Year Vegetarian Diet in Rheumatoid Arthritis." *Journal of the American Medical Association* (February 5, 1992), pp. 646–48.

Michael Rothfeld. *"Fasting: Are the Health Benefits Fact or Fiction?" The Detox Diet,* Elson Haas, M.D., Celestial Arts, 1966.

Tom Deters, D.C. "Should You Fast?" *Muscle & Fitness* (July 1995), pp. 94–95.

CHAPTER 5: PURIFYING BODY AND SPIRIT

Royce Flippin. "Breathe Easy: 6 Steps to Banishing Stress." *American Health* (July 1995), pp. 58–61.

Pam Grout. *Jumpstart Your Metabolism with the Power of Breath.* Patootie Press, 1996.

Lucy Lidell. *The Sensual Body.* (New York: Fireside Books, 1987), pp. 44–53, 56, and 70–74.

"The Benefits of Massage." *Better Homes and Gardens* (April 1991), pp. 55–58.

"Relax the Flash." *Prevention* (March 1993).

"Rub Out Asthma." *Prevention* (July 1995), p. 23.

Daryn Eller. "Please Touch! The Healing Power of Massage." *Redbook* (February 1995), pp. 66–68.

"Detox with Reflexology." *First* (April 1, 1996), pp. 20–21.

Laura Norman. *Feet First.* (New York: Fireside, 1988).

Nancy Arnott. "The Amazing Benefits of Massage." *Woman's World* (March 19, 1996), p. 26.

Michael Rothfeld. "Healing Touch." pp. 54–56.

"Hot Stuff." *Architectural Record* (April 1992), pp. 38 (2).

Fact sheets from Finneleo Sauna and Steam.

"Sauna Making You Sweat?" Internet: http://www/hotwired.com/drweil.

Ear coning instruction sheet. The Coning Company.

Jo Plane. "The A-Z of Water." Internet: http://balance.net/Eoo2o/.

Cheryl Solimini. "Let's Get Physical," *Country Living's Healthy Living,* pp. 80–82.

Peter Jaret. "Exercise to Beat the Blues." *Health* (November–December 1995), pp. 85–88.

Paul McCarthy. "Exercise and the Big C." *American Health* (March 1992), p. 121.

"Fitness Matters." *Better Homes and Gardens* (November 1991), pp. 63–64.

"Exercise May Prevent Cancer." *Time* (February 29, 1988).

Daryl Eller. "Exercises in Tranquility." *Essence* (January 1995), p. 67.

"Simple Steps to Inner Peace." *Woman's World* (April 30, 1996), p. 17.

"Meditation Prevents Panic Attacks." *American Health* (July–August 1996), p. 95.

Nancy Arnott. "The Relaxation Break That Can Add Years to Your Life." *Woman's World* (September 10, 1996), p. 44.

"Using the Relaxation Response." *Consumer Reports* (February 1993).

CHAPTER 6: COMPLETE YOUR DETOX: CREATE A SAFE HAVEN AND A NATURAL HOME SPA

David Steinman, and R. Michael Wisner. "Detoxify Your Life." *Let's Live* (November 1996), pp. 45–47.

"Cleaning the Air: Eliminate Indoor Air Pollution." *Green Living* (Winter 1995–96), pp. 22–26.

Jennifer Chrebet. "Is Your Office Making You Sick?" *American Health* (July–August 1996), pp. 92–94.

"Styrene in Foods: What Does It Mean?" *Science News* (September 17, 1994), p. 191.

"Seven Pampering Spa Treats for Next to Nothing." *Woman's World* (August 20, 1996), pp. 8–9.

"Wrinkle Remedies." *Natural Health* (March–April 1996), p. 164.

"Kitchen Apothecary." *Self* (August 6, 1996), p. 165.

Janice Cox. *Natural Beauty at Home* (New York: Henry Holt, 1995).

Pamela Boyer. "Bathing Beautifully." *Prevention* (June 1995), pp. 124–27.

Paula Begoun. "From the Neck Down: Soaking Your Cares Away," Knight-Ridder/Tribune News Service, December 8, 1994, p. 120.

"Six Skin Savers: Scrubs, Smoothers, and Steams." *Natural Health* (July–August), p. 82.

"Skin Scrubs You Can Make." *Health* (November–December 1995), p. 34.

"Some Serious Sloughing." *Natural Health* (March–April), p. 118.

CHAPTER 7: A GUIDE TO NATURAL, NUTRITIONAL PURIFIERS

Jensen Bernard, M.D. *Foods that Heal* (New York: Avery, 1963).

Nutrition Search Inc. *Nutrition Almanac.* (New York: McGraw-Hill, 1973).

Louise Frazier. *Louise's Leaves* (Bio-Dynamic Farming and Gardening Assoc., 1994).

Nancy Arnott. "Cures from Your Kitchen." *Woman's World* (March 26, 1996), p. 26.

Victoria Dolby. "The Women's Guide to Minerals." *The Nutrition Alert* (Nutrition Communications).

Betty Kamen, Ph.D. "Green Foods: Splendor in the Grass." *Let's Live* (September 1995), pp. 58–60.

"Yams Help Keep Menopause at Bay." *Woman's World* (May 7, 1996), p. 43.

"Nutrition Notes." *Health* (March–April 1996), p. 40.

"Think Zinc." *Healthnews* (August 6, 1996), p. 5.

Lambeth Hochwald. "Special-Interest Supplements." *Health* (July–August 1996), pp. 103–14.

Nancy Arnott. "Spice Your Way to a Long Healthy Life!" *Woman's World* (April 9, 1996), p. 26.

"Folic Acid: Vital to Your Vitality." *Parade Weekend* (August 2–4, 1996), p. 10.

William I. Young. "Staying Healthy: Spice up Your Life." *Los Angeles Sentinel* (March 22, 1995).

Liz Applegate. "Mother Nature's 'Superfoods'." *Runner's World* (March 3, 1995), p. 24.

Index